My painkiller Vipassana Meditation

My way out of the pain prison with 20 years intense meditation

Philip Popp

My painkiller Vipassana Meditation

2nd edition, paperback 11/2024

Editing: Gerd König
Cover Design: Philip Popp

ISBN: 9798346056447

DEDICATION

I dedicate this book to all people with chronic pain and hope that it will help and encourage some people.

CONTENTS

**The most difficult time in our lives is the best
opportunity to develop inner strength.**

Dalai Lama (*1935), ("The Smile of Heaven"), actually
Tenzin Gyatso, 14th spiritual and political leader of the
Tibetans, awarded the Nobel Peace Prize in 1989

FOREWORD

Have you ever been locked up? Maybe in a room or in an elevator? Then you probably know that oppressive feeling. And have you ever been in prison? Maybe you've taken a tour of a museum in an old prison or visited someone who was incarcerated. Can you imagine what that would be like? Let's say: what it would be like to sit in a small cell for four years?
My cell was tiny and gloomy, and over the years it had become smaller and smaller. My prison had no bars and no windows, and yet there was no escape. My prison was also invisible to most people. The walls of my cell were the dull, never-ending pain that accompanied my every waking moment. And my prison guards were my own thoughts, my fear and my anger. They fed off the pain and grew through it. Or was it the other way around? Only when I slept did I forget that I was locked up.

Again and again I asked myself how I had got into it. What crime had I committed? Would I ever be free again?
At the age of 18, I had a snowboarding accident with whiplash injuries and developed chronic neck and headaches as a result. My wild lifestyle at the time probably also played a role in this chronic pain. The constant pain gradually reduced my quality of life. A downward spiral was set in motion that eventually became a vicious circle.

Depressive thoughts and anxiety slowly crept into my life and gradually became a constant companion. Their power increased from day to day. It got so bad that panic attacks severely restricted my everyday life. As a result, I avoided many everyday situations that are normal for others and hid from life in my prime. I constantly felt like I was trapped in my own mind, and was desperately looking for a way out.

I had four years of unsuccessful and frustrating visits to the doctor and therapies behind me when I took my first Vipassana mediation course. It only took four days there before I got the impression that this type of meditation could support me and, with years of training, perhaps even help me out of this pain prison.

This impression seemed to be confirmed! When I completed my first full Vipassana course six months later, an extremely powerful change took place that shook and touched me to my core. After the two-week course, the usual panic attacks disappeared almost completely from my life and the intensity of the pain was suddenly reduced by a third. I was also able to move my neck much better again, which otherwise only had limited mobility due to the tension. After each subsequent meditation retreat, the pain decreased by a few more percent. And even in everyday life, daily practice helped me to reduce my pain levels, clear my confused head and cope with all the negative feelings associated with my chronic pain condition.

I mainly used meditation as a tool against my pain. A good meditation session reduced the pain many times better and more effectively than one or even several strong painkillers. As a result, I was able to cope with my everyday life much better again by meditating extensively every day.
I managed to complete my business studies in this way and have been working successfully as a consultant for business software ever since. In my worst years, I would never have dreamed that this would be possible. Before I discovered

meditation, I never expected that I would ever be able to do a "normal" job.

Furthermore, it was an enormous help to overcome the negative emotions, to deal with them more skillfully and finally to throw them out of the system. My fears gradually diminished and my self-confidence grew at the same time.

With this book, I would like to use my story to give an impression of how Vipassana meditation can help people and what changes it can bring about. In my opinion, it has a tremendous positive transformative power. However, it takes time and work. Nowadays, almost everyone knows that there are countless scientific studies that prove the many positive effects of regular meditation on health and enjoyment of life. For most people interested in meditation, however, it is not really tangible how much time and effort you really have to invest in order to achieve noticeable results. In principle, it is also not easy to give an answer to this question, as personalities, abilities and life situations differ greatly from person to person.

From a Buddhist perspective, every person and every living being brings their own karma with them. However, as I have practiced intensively over a long period of 20 years and have spent an estimated ten thousand hours in meditation, my story can perhaps give you an idea of what changes are possible and realistic over what period of time within the framework of a Western lifestyle.

My wish with my book is to inspire you to practice Vipassana meditation with some intensity. I firmly believe that this is one of the best investments a person can make in their life - because it has fundamentally changed mine.

CHILDHOOD - A PERFECT WORLD ON THE FARM

Country life

Before my world turned into a dark dungeon, I had a fairly normal childhood and a thoroughly rebellious youth.

When I was born, my parents were 23 and 21 years old. They got married in the same year and also took out a large loan to build a house, a cowshed and a milking facility.

I was a sweet, bright, but also sensitive and probably rather introverted child. I was reserved towards strangers at first. As the first of four siblings, I grew up in a small village with just under 400 inhabitants on a dairy farm. My father was a passionate farmer and was completely absorbed in his profession. My mother was a sports and music teacher by profession. However, she only worked in this profession for a short time as she became a mother at an early age. My father had grown up in the village and had helped out on his father's farm from an early age. After finishing secondary school, he did an apprenticeship and became a master farmer. My mother had come from the Saarland via Bad Bramstedt to Dithmarschen on the west coast, as her father had taken over the position of dairy director in a small town. She then studied in Kiel for a few years and graduated as a teacher there.

Working on a farm was not a nine-to-five job. My father always worked a lot, 14 hours was not unusual. The cows also had to be looked after and milked at the weekend. My mother looked after the children, did the bookkeeping and fed the calves.

Sometimes she also helped with milking or other work on the farm. She also looked after her horse. She generally had a wide range of interests and was particularly fond of music, horse riding and sport. But she also read a lot of novels, loved to talk, had a confident manner and loved to spend hours on the phone with friends and acquaintances. Both my father and my mother enjoyed going to birthday parties with their circle of friends, which consisted mainly of farmers and their wives. While my father liked to celebrate with alcohol and became more communicative and relaxed as a result, my mother didn't drink at all and was able to have a good time without it.

The farm, the high loan, all the work and the children were a great challenge and a dream come true at the same time. My mother had a big heart and usually generously overlooked the mistakes of others. She usually behaved very lovingly and warmly. Sometimes, however, she developed outbursts of anger that I was afraid of. And they were unpredictable. It wasn't necessarily because we children had done something seriously wrong. It was more a case of small mistakes slowly adding up. And when our mother's cup of tea overflowed at some point, the tension was released in an outburst of anger. Even the smallest mistake could then be a catastrophe. It was difficult for me to predict and made me feel insecure again and again. I loved my mother very much, but sometimes I was also afraid of her anger.

My parents had the usual division of responsibilities at that time. My mother was responsible for the household and the children and my father primarily took care of the farm. He was a very determined and hard-working farmer who responsibly ensured that his family was financially secure. Although he was warm-hearted by nature and strived for harmony, the amount of work he did often led to tensions, as I unfortunately didn't share his passion for farming. I also enjoyed playing outside in the sandpit or on the yard, but I enjoyed sitting in the living room and watching TV just as much.

My father worked a lot and demanded a lot from himself and his body. Perhaps a little too much at times. From the age of 30, he gradually developed various allergies and food intolerances, which made life and work more difficult for him. He consulted various doctors and underwent examinations and therapies, but these could only help him to a limited extent. At some point, he could only tolerate contact with the animals to a limited extent, as he had also developed a severe allergy to animal hair with asthma. As a result, the farm got an employee to take over some of the milking to relieve my father.

Back then, my life mainly consisted of table tennis, playing computer games and fishing. I had been attending grammar school for a year. However, as most of my classmates were more than 10 kilometers away, I usually went to my best friend Matthias' house after school and we played various business simulations or soccer managers on his C64 all day. My favorite game was Vermeer. In the game, you had to prove yourself as a landowner and art connoisseur. You managed coffee, cocoa and tobacco plantations and used the proceeds to buy works of art at auctions. You had to be careful not to get hold of a fake. You played Vermeer all day, then you could save your score and continue playing the next day. Sometimes a game lasted for days. I was fascinated by building up these strategic business ventures.

Table tennis junkie

I practiced table tennis three to four times a week. On Tuesdays and Wednesdays I played at our club and on Thursday at the district base training in Meldorf, where I also went to school. Later on, we even drove almost as far as Elmshorn, which was around 60 kilometers away, to the district training base every week. At the weekends, I usually took part in matches with my team or we went to tournaments with Harry and Wiebke. Harry and Wiebke were my uncle and aunt, who had also coached me in table tennis since I was six. They invested a lot of their free time traveling with children and young people to point games and tournaments. I often brought home medals and occasionally a trophy.

I actually got on well with my table tennis and team colleagues. Nevertheless, the children in the table tennis club often teased me because I lived on a farm. Sometimes they called me Hinnerk, sometimes they said I smelled like a cowshed, and on various occasions they made nasty comments. I didn't take this teasing well at all, I didn't have a thick skin, I reacted quite sensitively and felt hurt. Sometimes I cursed the fact that I lived on a farm. I was constantly expected to help out on the farm and I was also teased and criticized by other children because of it. Why couldn't my father be a doctor or a teacher?

In the fresh air

On many days I went fishing with my friend Matthias on nearby meadows and ditches. We often even fished overnight and camped on the bank. It was always a challenge for us to find the right spot, the right bait and the right time to land an eel or a pike. Our biggest fishing project consisted of our own pond, which I built together with Matthias behind the fence of our garden.

It took us several days to dig a hole that was three meters long and 1.80 meters deep. In the process, I got several blisters on my hands and developed thick calluses. We lined the pond with two layers of silage tarpaulin, of which my father had plenty lying around the yard. I even managed to persuade him to let me have a piece of new tarpaulin. First we collected aquatic plants from the surrounding ditches in the marsh, the nearby biotope and the village pond and then filled the pond with water. Next, we used the landing net to catch tadpoles and water striders from the village pond. Finally, small fish such as roach and small eels were added, which could be seen swimming in the pond with a little patience and an attentive eye. One day, when we saw a heron flying away from the kitchen window, I was outraged that it had dared to help itself to our pond.

Favorite series

If there was any free time left - and it seemed to me that there was far too much of it - I continued to watch TV often. As long as I wasn't playing computer games all day, I watched at least three hours of TV a day. My favorite series was A Colt for All Seasons with Colt Seavers. In the series, he played a stuntman who worked as a bounty hunter on the side. Together with his good-looking assistant Jody and his cousin, the clumsy pretty boy Howie, they hunted down fugitive defendants. He performed all kinds of adventurous stunts with his pick-up truck. Colt Seavers was the hero of my childhood and early youth, and I wanted to be a stuntman like him when I grew up.

The daily Star Trek episode that was broadcasted every afternoon and at weekends was also almost sacred to me. I was fascinated by the utopian future technologies such as beaming, wormholes and warp-space Drives as well as the different intergalactic forms of aliens. Every day on TV I saw Lieutenant Worf from the Klingons - a proud, emotional and warlike civilization. I was also fascinated by Spock, who belonged to the Vulcans. They had very high moral standards based on pure logic. Emotions and selfish behavior were alien to them. Then there was the android Lieutenant Data, who was a human-like machine based on artificial intelligence. There were also many other exciting types and technologies.

The whole Star Trek universe was a great inspiration for me. As my parents weren't particularly strict when it came to television, I was already watching formative films such as Star Wars, Rambo and Rocky at a relatively young age. I also watched some of them with my siblings out of habit or boredom, perhaps also for the company. Then I consumed everything that could be seen on our five channels at the time. From Night Rider to A-Team and MacGyver to Lindenstraße and Gute Zeiten, schlechte Zeiten.

I also loved watching sports broadcasts. Whenever there was an Olympic Games, I spent every spare minute in front of the TV watching all kinds of sports.

Back to milking cows

As our family ran a dairy farm, my father milked the cows twice a day, seven days a week. The animals seemed to me to be quite sensitive when it came to milking on time, because my father always got nervous if there was a delay on a trip to the zoo or a visit to friends and acquaintances. A day out with us usually only started after my father had milked the cows in the morning. had already milked and fed her. And we had to be back in time for the same procedure to be repeated in the evening. So an outing could only take place between 9am and 4pm. We therefore never went on family outings lasting several days and never went on family vacations, which I always envied other children for.

Computer fascination

For my twelfth birthday, my parents gave me a second-hand Amiga 500, a personal computer with which you could play games similar to those on my friend Matthias' C64. Only the Amiga was more advanced, had more memory and more computing power and the games were more graphically sophisticated than the C64. I spent a lot of time alone in front of the computer playing Soccer Manager or Indiana Jones. This was an adventure role-playing game in which you had to find artifacts in the role of an adventurous archaeologist. You had to solve puzzles and complete tasks in various countries, continents and game scenes in order to find valuable objects - before the Nazis, who were also looking for them. Pirates was another favorite game of mine. You started with a ship in the Caribbean and chose one of four nationalities. You could sail under the English, Spanish, Dutch or Portuguese flag or start as a pirate ship. The object of the game was to attack and plunder other ships, conquer cities in the Caribbean and add them to your flag. You traded goods and bought weapons to increase your firepower. You also forged clever alliances to increase your power and influence. With these games, I completely forgot about the time around me. Hours and whole days flew by. I was still playing with Matthias, who had meanwhile given his C64 to his brother and got an Amiga 500 himself. Sometimes we played at my place, sometimes at his. But since I went to grammar school in Meldorf and my friend went to secondary school in St. Michaelisdonn, we had grown apart a little. We no longer met up to play every day, but only once or twice a week.

The back pinches

When I was about 13, my mother often pricked me between the shoulder blades with her finger and said: "Keep it straight, otherwise your back will grow crooked!"

She had been doing this a lot for a while. Although it annoyed the hell out of me, I also had the feeling that I was slumping my shoulders a bit and not walking upright and straight. But it was more the aesthetic aspect that bothered me. However, it seemed to be a habitual posture and my mother's pricking didn't really help. However, as my back was also hurting more often at the same point, right in the middle between my shoulder blades, my mother sent me to our GP, who prescribed physiotherapy for my back.

From then on, I did exercises once a week with a physiotherapist. I rolled on a ball or lay on the floor and did strengthening exercises for my muscles. I was supposed to do these exercises regularly at home too. However, I didn't enjoy them and I could rarely bring myself to do them. Fortunately, the back pain eventually subsided all by itself.

YOUTH - FROM ONE PARTY TO THE NEXT

The Pantera concert

I had been going to grammar school for a few years by then and had been listening to heavy metal music for quite some time. I often wore T-shirts and hoodies from popular metal bands. I had also let my hair grow a little longer, as befitted a real metal fan. One day, I accompanied my school friend Jens home again and then his mother drove us to Hamburg. She dropped us off on the Reeperbahn at Große Freiheit, where the Pantera concert was taking place. We were really looking forward to the concert, as Pantera had been one of our favorite bands for some time. Their new album *"Far Beyond Driven"*, which they had released a few months ago, excited us both. As it would be a while before the band played, we drank a lot of beer and "Vodka-O" to warm up. When the metal band Pantera finally kicked off with a decent delay, the whole concert hall shook. There must have been almost 1000 visitors. The band produced a powerful sound and we enthusiastically "moshed" with the crowd right at the front. At the climax of the concert, we climbed onto the stage with a few daredevils and, for the first time in our lives did "Stage diving". Although there were minders who didn't like it at all, we didn't let them stop us. It felt phenomenal to jump into the crowd, to be caught by all those arms and to be carried weightlessly through the room. We walked around the Reeperbahn after the concert, drenched in sweat. The cold winter air made it uncomfortable, and as my cousin wouldn't pick us up until an hour later, we waited that long at Burger King and ate cheeseburgers. A couple of dolled-up prostitutes in thick bomber jackets walked in front of the entrance and Fanny packs up and down.

"This really is the depths of the red light district," I thought, feeling a little uncomfortable in this environment. Unlike me, Jens was an extrovert and always enjoyed talking to strangers. He quickly struck up a conversation with the guy at the next table, who was two or three years older than us and looked a bit run-down. I wasn't entirely comfortable with this, but as Jens had a good conversation with him, he joined us at the table. He told us that he liked smoking weed and Jens joined in the conversation with interest. The guy then told us that he had also smoked "Shore" before and asked us if we needed anything. We said no. I was delighted when we finally had to leave because my cousin Kai was supposed to pick us up by car in front of Davidswache at one o'clock. On the way there, Jens explained to me that 'shore' was another word for heroin, and a shiver ran down my spine out of anxiety.

"Hello you two! Well, was the concert good?" asked my cousin.

"Yes, super good! They had a great sound and we even did some stage diving!" I replied proudly.

"However, my ears are ringing quite a lot now. That was very loud."

On Monday at school, the whistling in my ears still accompanied the lessons. However, it didn't bother me too much, but reminded me of what a great concert we had experienced. It took a whole three days for the tinnitus to subside.

Disco fever

When I was 15, I liked to party regularly in the discos in the area. On Friday nights, I would go out with a few friends to the disco in Brunsbüttel; I wouldn't get home until two o'clock on those nights, really drunk. I slept until midday when my parents called me for lunch.

Still a little winded, I sat down at the kitchen table with the others, drowsy. I regularly managed to tip over my glass of milk and soak the whole table in milk. After a night of drinking, I was always a little restless in the morning. After lunch, I would listen to loud metal music in my room. Pantera, Biohazard and Fear Factory were some of my favorite bands. I regularly bought the magazines *Metalhammer* and *Rockhard*, and the posters from the magazines adorned the walls of my room. I invested some of my money in music CDs. Whereas two years previously I had mainly bought pop CDs, I was now listening to metal in different variations. My preference was not classic heavy metal, but rather hardcore, power and even some death metal.

I always prepared for the evening in the same way: First, I squeezed out the latest pimples and disinfected them with Clearasil. Then I shaved and tamed my hair with gel. Finally, I packed a bottle of Korn in my Bundeswehr rucksack. With my hair almost reaching my chin, I apparently looked older than I was. Because when I bought the Korn as a precaution during the week, I was rarely asked for my ID. If I was asked once, I showed it confidently and was usually let through anyway. Apparently the cashiers didn't look too closely or didn't feel like doing the math. In addition to the vodka, I also got two Tetra Paks of orange juice to mix.

In the late afternoon, I cycled the eight kilometers to my friend Kirsten's house in Meldorf. We cuddled up in her room and watched Beverly Hills 902010 the night before.

As the evening progressed, her sister Marianne and her gang, who were all two years older than us, came over. A friend of Kirsten's usually joined them too, and they all brought different types of alcohol and mixed drinks. Kirsten's small room was glowing with and we were soon pretty drunk. After all, we had a sizeable collection of sour apple, Blue Curacao, vodka, Korn and sparkling wine in stock and mixed it all with orange juice. If we started drinking heavily at these pre-parties, we got away with it more cheaply and didn't have to buy as many of the expensive drinks at the disco. And of course we also mixed a few bottles for the road. Then we set off.

Our regular disco was twenty kilometers away in a small village called Welmbüttel. It wasn't easy to get there. Sometimes a friend's parents drove us there, and we usually found a ride back. My parents were so cool that I could always call them if I couldn't get home otherwise - although I tried not to do that too often.

In Welmbüttel, they played metal and rock music like Rage Against the Machine or Nirvana. We moshed, played table football and continued drinking. To save money, we hid our self-mixed bottles outside behind the disco. We'd go out drinking in small groups from time to time. On the way back, I regularly had to concentrate very hard to avoid throwing up in the back seat.

For years, I led a wild, exciting lifestyle in this way. My circle of friends, which I thought was very cool, was mostly older. I had a great girlfriend and was constantly meeting new people at parties. Even after a night of drinking, I was quickly fit again and could party again the next day or play table tennis if I had point games or a tournament.

When drunk, I was eloquent and funny. In this state, I

could quickly make a connection with almost anyone and gain sympathy for myself; I was able to master almost any situation quite elegantly. This gave me enormous self-confidence, which I didn't have when I was sober. I liked myself when I was drunk!

When I was sober, it was completely different. Straight I often found it difficult to find the right words when talking to strangers or in unfamiliar situations. I often couldn't think of a good topic of conversation. Small talk had always been a horror for me. I preferred in-depth conversations or conversations about a specific topic that I knew a lot about. But luckily there was alcohol, which made life much more exciting, thrilling and easier.

The alcohol also acted like a protective armor. Without it, I felt easily attacked and insecure, and it was difficult to counter critical comments with a quick wit. After a few drinks, however, I felt protected against the nasty comments of others. They no longer bothered me at all. On the contrary: I fired back a volley at the same level and even had a lot of fun competing with my fellow human beings in this way - although I was always careful not to be mean and not to overshoot the mark - after all, I knew from my own experience how unpleasant that could be.

Kuden Open Air

On a hot, sunny afternoon, I was sitting with my friends on the edge of the football pitch in Wolmersdorf. We often met there at the weekend to play soccer. We played for a while and then planned the rest of the day. I was in a great mood because there was a big event coming up today. The Kuden Open Air was taking place on the same day: a rural youth event that attracts thousands of visitors every year. It had been great the previous year, an exhilarating experience.

The music wasn't exactly to my taste (too mainstream), but that didn't matter as I was able to meet lots of friends and acquaintances there and party excessively.

Everyone in our group wanted to go to this spectacle in the evening.

We talked about whose parents would be going. Most of us went to the grammar school in Meldorf, a small town with a population of 8,000. Most of my clique came from a small village nearby called Wolmersdorf; no one lived more than 200 meters away from anyone else. I envied them that, because in my village and the surrounding area there was no one I called a friend since I had grown increasingly estranged from my childhood best friend. At that time, Wolmersdorf was increasingly becoming my second home and the home base of our clique. That's where we met up, played soccer and had our first parties.

While the others didn't want to go to the open air until the evening, I couldn't wait that long. I knew that in weather like this, many people would be there from 12 noon, barbecuing and drinking. The party in the afternoon was the best, you couldn't miss it. So I said goodbye to my friends and walked to Meldorf, three kilometers away, to hitchhike from there to St. Michaelisdonn, another twelve kilometers away. I had an appointment there with a friend from the table tennis club. His mother would drive us to Kuden.

I felt well prepared for the open air. I had bought a bottle of Korn and pre-mixed it with two 1.5-liter bottles of Coke. I carried the two bottles loosely in my hands on the way to Meldorf and took a few sips from time to time as I walked. It was going to be a great party! Arriving in Meldorf, I positioned myself near the end of the town on the main road and held my thumb out to flag down a car. An Audi Quattro pulled up relatively quickly and let me in. I was lucky: the driver was able to take me straight to St.

Michaelisdonn. He was wearing white gloves, which seemed a bit surreal to me. On leaving the town, he accelerated so fast in his Quattro that I felt like I was at a rocket launch. What a blast! A good omen for the rest of the day, I decided. I felt great, full of anticipation for the party ahead. I arrived at my friend's house on time and his mother drove us to Kuden, a few kilometers away, together with another friend of his. It went like clockwork. The festival site stretched over several large fields and was already full of caravans, tents, tractors and cars. The whole area was a hive of activity.

We looked for a place to pitch our tent and met a number of friends who were all in a great mood. Some of them were buzzed and some were already quite drunk. We had our first corn mixture and set up the tent. One or two mixtures later, we started a tour around the grounds.

I knew that Isa and Nele from my school would also be there in the afternoon and wanted to camp there. As I had liked Isa for some time, we went off to look for them. We soon found them sitting in front of their tent and joined them. They were already a bit buzzed and we were fooling around and having a good time together. Parties like that were great. I completely forgot about time, just went for it, and sooner or later I always met someone. Even if you only knew each other briefly, on such a glorious sunny day and with a lot of alcohol, you quickly got talking and soon knew each other better. Since I had started partying and going to parties or discos every weekend, my life had definitely become more exciting. Whereas I used to spend most of my free time playing table tennis or computer games, this had now changed completely. It was party time at the weekend. I had also been single again for a few months. I'd broken up with my ex-girlfriend because I'd fallen for another girl. It hadn't worked out the way I had imagined. But life was great, I had lots of friends, was popular and enjoyed good chances at the girls.

The afternoon passed quickly. Before the evening was over, I had met countless acquaintances, got to know new people, talked to nice girls and drunk a lot of alcohol. After my two mixed grain bottles were empty, all kinds of people had offered me all sorts of hard alcohol and I had accepted most of them gratefully. In the meantime, I had lost sight of Isa and Nele without any kind of approach. By now it was dark and everything was getting a bit hazy. I had found a full pack of cigarettes and was so drunk that I lit one without thinking about it. As soon as I'd smoked it, I lit another one.

That probably did me in, because I didn't normally smoke cigarettes. While I was walking around the campsite smoking one moment, the next I found myself in the dark. I didn't know where I was and I was shivering. There was a kind of membrane around me. I felt trapped. Only after a while did I realize that I was in a tent. I felt nauseous and I suspected that I must have had a film rupture. I was also totally disoriented. Fortunately, there were friends of mine outside the tent who were soon picked up by their parents. They looked after me and even drove me home. I didn't know what time it was and didn't bother giving it a second thought. In my state, I even managed to lock the front door behind me - probably because my father had warned me some time ago to lock the door at night if I came home late. Then I stumbled up the stairs, threw myself on the bed in my clothes and immediately dozed off.

At some point, I was woken up by heavy knocking noises. At first I didn't understand where they were coming from, until I realized

that someone was knocking on my window. But that couldn't actually be. My room was on the top floor of our house. I finally realized that my father was standing on a ladder in front of my window, banging on the window quite vehemently and bawling loudly. I staggered downstairs, still completely drunk and also sleepy, and went to the front door. When I saw my parents standing in front of the door, I realized that I had locked them out. They must have come home after me. As a reward for letting them in, my father slapped me hard on the face. I hadn't been prepared for that; it only happened very rarely. Had it ever happened before? Why? Was it because they had been waiting outside for so long, or because I was so drunk at the age of 16, which was probably not appropriate for a 16-year-old? Probably both, I speculated. If I had been sober, I would definitely have been pretty shocked, as the attack was violent and unexpected. In my state, however, I just staggered up the stairs to my bed in a daze and went back to sleep.

Soon afterwards, or so it seemed to me, I was startled out of my sleep and saw my Uncle Harry standing in front of me in my room. "Hello Philip, did you oversleep? You've got district rankings today. Nils is downstairs in the car waiting," he said.

"Oh shit, shit, yeah, I overslept, I'll hurry up," I replied. I was still feeling sick as a dog as I packed my table tennis gear in record time. I had completely forgotten that I was supposed to play table tennis today. It was actually an important thing, the district ranking. If I was in great form, I definitely had a chance of playing at the top and possibly even qualifying for the state ranking list.

In the end, I didn't play too badly despite my terrific hangover. I was a bit shaky and couldn't eat until the afternoon, but at least I didn't embarrass myself and even won a few games.

However, I didn't manage to qualify for the state ranking list. But I didn't think that was a bad thing, because I had had a fantastic party yesterday. I had no regrets!

Fight with mom

While I had previously put up with my mother's occasional outbursts of anger and usually ended up cowering, I now tended to counter them more. As a result, the arguments escalated more and more violently. When I had once again celebrated properly and slept until midday, my mother came stomping into my room angrily and pulled up the outside blinds: "Well, have you slept in yet? While you're sleeping here until noon, your father and I are already working hard for many hours so that you children have a good life! And you're making a lazy living here at our expense. What do you say to that?"

'Oh man, what's she been up to now?' I thought, blinded by the sudden brightness as I struggled to get up in bed. '"You're barely awake before you get hit on the head! I replied aloud, no less defiantly: 'Good morning. I got home late, so I sleep late, of course. That doesn't mean I'm lazy at your expense! I help out a lot, I drive the tractor, mow the lawn and help out around the farm."

"We had agreed that you would clean up here in the attic every two weeks, vacuum and clean the bathroom. When was the last time you did that?"

"Yes, that was a while ago," I admitted. "But we had also said that this should be my job instead of helping out on the farm. Because I wanted to do something inside rather than outside. And I've done a few things recently

outside, I helped drive the straw and seal the silage clamp. I think I help out quite a lot."

"So, do you think so? Have you ever looked at how many other boys your age from the village help out on their farms?" my mother asked in a sharp tone. "And when Dad asks you if you can help, you walk around all day with a sour face. He doesn't even like to ask you anymore!"

"It was your decision to buy a farm! That's not what I want to do! I'm only ever supposed to help out! Am I just a worker for you? When does Dad ever have time and interest for me? Has Dad ever come to one of my table tennis tournaments and watched? No! Nils' parents do that all the time, by the way. And about helping out: When I look at my friends, they don't have to help their fathers in the doctor's surgery or teach in the classroom with their father!" I replied defiantly.

My mother's voice became more and more energetic: "If you carry on like this, always partying and living for the day, you won't become anything sensible, or do you see it differently?"

"I don't want to have a great job. I don't need a lot of money and it's enough for me if I can live on welfare later. The main thing is that I have time to hang out with my friends and can do whatever I feel like doing. And by the way, I don't want to be older than 40 anyway! Life is boring as an adult, you're already half dead! You work hard during the day in a boring job. In the evening you're so exhausted that all you can do is watch TV and you rarely see your friends. And apart from that, you constantly have the kids on your back and have to put your own pleasure on the back burner."

"Go on like that, friend," my mother hissed

angrier. She left the room, slammed the door and I heard her stomping loudly down the stairs.

These arguments became more and more frequent and heated, and our relationship deteriorated further with every argument.

Stoned in Wolmersdorf

I often rode my bike to Wolmersdorf in the afternoon. My

first port of call was my friends Davids' or Jens' home. If I couldn't find anyone there, I simply asked their parents where everyone was. Everything was just a stone's throw away from each other. It wasn't unusual for us to get ten players on the pitch for soccer. In the afternoons, we watched TV and smoked pot, played skat and smoked pot or played Playstation and smoked pot. The most popular game was Bomberman, because you could play it with four players against each other at the same time and you could still manage it even when you were extremely stoned. Most of the time we smoked bong, a kind of water pipe. It was cheaper because a bong head was much wider than taking a few drags on a joint. You could also blow the smoke out of the window, so the room wasn't quite so smoky. When you smoked a joint in the room, everything smelled incredibly like hash or weed.

Towards the evening, we started to pre-party. We turned up the music and got into the mood with beer, vodka or whisky mixes or even wine. Later, we usually went to a party, disco or open-air event. I always liked the pre-party phase the best. We were still in a relatively small, intimate group, and as the alcohol consumption increased, so did the atmosphere and volume.

When I was 16, I experienced the summer of my life. That year, most of my friends bought a Deutsche Bahn summer vacation ticket. For only 15 marks

you could spend the whole summer vacation driving all over Schleswig-Holstein and even as far as Hamburg or Sylt. I got ten grams of Polle from a friend in the neighboring village. This is a yellowish, particularly resinous hashish. I had been with Thea for five months and was madly in love. Like the majority of our core clique, she also lived in Wolmersdorf. We went to Sylt with a group of people almost every other day and spent the day on the beach. We'd get out the water bong on the train and fill up the whole six-person compartment. I had built a bong out of a gray drainpipe. It didn't look particularly nice, but it worked well, and at least it was homemade. By my standards at the time, everything was going perfectly: I was with the girl of my dreams, had lots of friends around me and enjoyed the time we all spent together. We all thought it was cool that we were usually stoned. It was part of our clique's lifestyle. It always had a strong effect on me. After a bong head, I was often so flat that I didn't check much. When we were stoned, we called it "being flat" or "being wide". When I was wide, I always thought the others were looking at me. Sometimes that was paranoia. A bit of paranoia was part of the flash. However, I often got such puffy, red eyes that it actually showed. My brain felt so turned upside down that I could no longer understand normal connections until the effect had subsided to some extent.

It was almost impossible for me to talk to my parents about any organizational matters when I was heavily stoned. I preferred to stay out of their way. With the others, I always admired the fact that they were still able to have a reasonably normal conversation with adults. I then found it difficult just to talk; I simply didn't know what to say. The impressions from the intoxication were far too blatant and intense for me to

could have put into words. This effect was of course stupid when you were in a group of people. Fortunately, it could be mitigated by drinking alcohol.

The first pain

Three weeks after school started again, everything changed. Thea had been acting differently for weeks. When she finally started to distance herself, I slowly realized that I was probably clinging and that was why she was withdrawing. Nothing was more pathetic than clinging! So I gave her the distance she seemed to need. We met less often, talked less on the phone. I was afraid it might end. I stopped saying "I love you" just to see if she would say it first at some point. But nothing happened. After all, we hadn't seen each other for six days - an eternity for me. I wanted to be with her every minute of my life.

It had been seven days since I had heard from Thea. I sat in math class for the first two lessons and couldn't concentrate on anything. I knew that Thea had a double lesson in biology and had to come by our room afterwards. During the big break, I intercepted her and said in a shaky voice: "You haven't been in touch for the last few days, and before that you kept your distance. I need to know this now, I can't take it anymore or I'll go crazy. It feels like you want to break up with me. Is that the case?"

She replied somewhat hesitantly: "Yes, you're probably right, it doesn't really feel like love to me anymore. I don't think it makes sense anymore. I'm sorry."

There was nothing more to say. I turned around without another word and went out into the schoolyard.

I tried very hard to pull myself together and not break down in tears. As I had dropped French, I was now the only one with two free periods. I was alone in the schoolyard and cursed life. My world had collapsed. I only felt pain and misery inside me. My head was empty. I had never felt like this before! Without Thea, everything no longer made sense. Even though we had only been a couple for six months, I had felt more fulfilled and alive with her than ever before. I would have loved to spend my whole life with her. Now it was all over in one fell swoop!

I couldn't do any homework for the next two months. As soon as I sat down on my own, thoughts of her flashed through my mind and tormented me, making me sad, mad and panicky. This is how a heroin junkie in withdrawal must feel! I couldn't bear to be without her. My heart was broken and it wasn't going to be mended any time soon, if that was even possible. For a while, I didn't even care that I got in trouble from the teachers for missing homework. What difference did it make? Was that bad? Was it important? Not if you put it in relation to the pain I was feeling.

The teaching of karma

In eleventh grade, I chose philosophy instead of religion as an elective subject because I found the famous ancient Greek philosophers such as Socrates and Plato exciting. However, I didn't get on particularly well with the teacher and found the lessons boring. I wasn't as enthusiastic as I had hoped. That's why I switched back to religious education after the first semester. I liked the teacher there, but we first dealt with the subject of biblical exegesis, i.e. researching different editions of the Bible.

Unfortunately, I also found it bland and dry. But when we got to know other religions, I was still glad that I had changed subjects.

When we were studying Hinduism, I heard about the concept of rebirth and karma for the first time. At first it seemed absurd to me that people in our modern age believed in rebirth and karma. But the more I learned about it, the more I became fascinated by the idea and the religion. There was not just one god in Hinduism, but a multitude of gods. Next, we went through Buddhism, and rebirth and karma came up as topics there too. Here, however, there was the Buddha, who sought and achieved salvation from the cycle of rebirths around 2500 years ago in India with the help of deep meditation. This religion also fascinated me, although I did not understand why the

Buddha did not want to be reborn. As I understood it, one actually wanted to live on and not die. So it could only be desirable to be reborn. We then went on to discuss Islam. I also found it interesting, but I wasn't that fascinated by it.

In twelfth grade, I painted a big red OM, the symbol of Hinduism, on my winter jacket so that it couldn't be overlooked. The symbol had an attractive effect on me. I thought it was pretty and also enjoyed the fact that most people probably couldn't relate to the symbol. When my rebellious nature came to the fore even more a few months later, I also painted my white and blue training jacket with the words "Fuck you" in thick red lettering. Anyone I turned my back on could now read that in big letters.

The first Goa party

As so often, we were sitting in Jörg's small room one evening. It was shrouded in mysterious black light and crammed with computer technology and accessories such as lava lamps and didgeridoos. This time the group was small: Jens, Jörg, our host, Florian and my new girlfriend Isa. We pre-partied and mentally prepared ourselves for our first Goa open air party. Shortly before midnight, we all set off together in Jörg's car towards Rendsburg and arrived at the festival site three quarters of an hour later. I was amazed at the size of the staked-out parking lot in the middle of nowhere, and we looked for a spot on the stubble field.

First of all, we made ourselves comfortable with a blanket near the car. Some distance away, we could already hear the booming bass of the music. We smoked with the small, handy acrylic bong that I had bought a few months ago. I smoked two heads of hash and tobacco, and was pretty high afterwards. Then we made our way towards the music. I was amazed when I saw the swirling crowd of people - shrouded in artificial fog and black light - moving to the beat of the music. It was an impressive spectacle to see thousands of people stomping and moving ecstatically to the psychedelic music - most of them in a unique dance style that I had never seen before. The atmosphere and flair of the scene fascinated and inspired me immediately.

After letting off steam on the dance floor for a while, we explored the many stalls that had gathered around the open-air area together. There were food stalls offering exotic Indian dishes such as lentil curry or chai tea. The food stalls mostly consisted of a tent with a chill-out area, which was carefully carpeted. People sat in the chill-out area, smoking weed, eating, chatting or just chilling out. Everything had a very exotic touch,

which I found extremely attractive. Then there were various stalls where you could buy tie-dyed hippie clothing or scarves, as well as some stalls with pipes, bongs and other paraphernalia that covered the usual stoner needs. I was enchanted by this world and marveled at everything I had never seen before.

I also enjoyed moving to these deep basses with their wild, psychedelic sounds. After some time on the dance floor, I entered a trance-like state and forgot everything else around me. It was less about dancing together and more about getting into a special state through dancing, where you were completely in the moment. Suddenly there was only the movement and the music. The high from smoking weed made the music and the dance experience even more intense and gave the whole thing a special spice. It wasn't until the early hours of the morning that we made our way home, happy and enriched by this new experience.

Shivamoon with mushrooms

A few months later, we went to Shivamoon in Mecklenburg-Vorpommern for a weekend. This was one of the biggest Goa open air festivals in Germany with about 20,000 visitors. This time, we were a larger group of over ten friends. After a four-hour drive, we set up our tents in the early evening in good spirits and with a cold beer in our hands. When someone passed by our camp and offered us Mexican mushrooms, I bought three grams and shared them with a friend.

That was the first time I had taken mushrooms. My friend already had some experience. He explained to me that one and a half grams was exactly the right dose for the first time, as it was not too high, but enough to give me a good feeling

Flash. After half an hour to an hour, I noticed that there was a change. Friends of mine who had taken mushrooms before had warned me that a mushroom trip could cause nausea and you might vomit.

Fortunately, I was spared that. Instead, I realized that my perception was slowly changing. Everything suddenly looked so interesting! The colors and the lights had a strange fascination for me. People, but also the lights and simply everything looked and felt so much more loving than usual. I felt a pleasant connection with everything around me. I had the feeling that I had reached another level of consciousness where the world felt new. I made my way to the dance floor and danced to the booming Goa music. Focusing on the psychedelic elements of the music, I felt myself merging with the music in that moment, which was disturbing and uplifting at the same time. The intoxication of the senses and colors lasted for several hours, and I felt happy and relaxed the next day as well.

The allure of intoxication

Smoking weed had been part of my life since I was 16. For me, it was part of a kind of modern hippie lifestyle that I identified with. We were a big clique of 20 to 30 people who all smoked weed more or less often, and I felt at home in this clique. It was like my second family. It was probably even more important than my real family for a while.

Smoking weed became more and more a part of clique life. Whether we were hanging out at a swimming lake in summer, sitting at someone's house in winter and playing Playstation or skat, someone usually had something to smoke with them.

When I was wide, time felt different. It passed slower. I perceived everything more intensely. Tastes, music, colors and touch left a stronger impression. My senses seemed to be much more sensitive. I found this extremely pleasant in many situations, for example when listening to music or eating. Sometimes I got a real feeding frenzy. Stoned, even brushing my teeth could be an exciting sensory experience.

But sometimes it was also unpleasant. If you went to a place with lots of people while stoned, you risked total sensory overload because your perception was far too sensitive. I also felt like my thoughts were getting louder. When I smoked a bong head, I felt catapulted into the present. In this state, I was more frugal, didn't need so much action, would rather chill out than do something, would rather watch a movie than talk too much.

But sometimes I was also overwhelmed by all the information, perceptions and feelings that were flooding into me so intensely. I often had the impression that very powerful feelings were rising up from deep within me, from my subconscious. Sometimes I was unable to think clearly or have a sensible conversation for hours. In such a state, I had to be careful where I went because I couldn't cope with all situations in this state.

Inspired by a friend, I tried my hand at growing a few cannabis plants. He had given me cannabis seeds and I planted them in small pots and grew them on the windowsill. Small plants grew up and I enjoyed watching them. I already felt like a little hobby gardener. In the morning, before I went to school, I would put them on the east side in front of the bathroom skylight. When I came back from school, I positioned them in the passageway room on the west side so that the sun would provide them with some direct light throughout the day.

After the first two plants shot up and became bushier, I planted two of them outside in a nice spot where they were protected but also got plenty of sun. While one didn't really develop, the other grew 2.30 meters high due to the exceptionally hot and sunny summer and produced an enormous number of flowers. The stem developed woody and reached a diameter of over five centimeters. The cannabis plant produced lots of potent, resinous flowers. Thanks to the sunny summer of the century, I now had a fantastic amount of weed available for my own consumption. I could make do with it for a long time. I no longer had to make any effort to organize hashish and I also saved a lot of money. When I was at home in the evenings during the week, I usually watched TV with my parents in the living room until nine and then went upstairs. I would often smoke a bong head in my room and blow the smoke out of the window. Then I would spend a few hours stoned in my room watching TV, reading books or playing computer games. I usually fell asleep late because I wanted to experience and enjoy the pleasant, different state of consciousness for longer. As a result, I usually didn't get enough sleep and struggled to get up the next morning. I felt groggy. I missed my school bus almost twice a week. Then I hitchhiked to school and was usually 10 to 15 minutes late for lessons. I often spent the evenings during the week with friends, where smoking weed was often on the agenda.

SNOWBOARD ACCIDENT AND DREADLOCKS - THE BEGINNING OF THE END OF THE PARTY

Ski vacation in Austria

We had taken the back of the "youth bus" that was taking my friends and me on a ski trip to Austria. We consumed a considerable amount of beer on the outward journey. Some of us even dared to smoke bongs secretly, bent behind the back of the seat in front of us. They tried to keep the smoke in their lungs for as long as possible so that most of it was absorbed and as little as possible came out again and smoked out the bus. They blew the last of it into a pillow and then opened the tilting windows for a while. Nevertheless, it was obvious that sooner or later one of the adults was bound to smell it. But to my surprise, nothing much happened apart from a small warning.

I myself had my small water bong and three grams of hash with me. As most of the others carried much larger quantities, it should be enough for ten days. I also always got stoned pretty quickly, so I never needed much. Many of my friends consumed much larger quantities than I did, and

I was always amazed at how they still managed to get on with their lives reasonably well.

It was the fourth time that I went on a skiing vacation with the Meldorf sports club to the large youth hostel in St. Michael in Austria over Easter. Our group consisted of around 150 people in three large buses. A large part of our group took part in the trip, including my friend Isa, who I had been dating for a few months now. Her mother organized together

with her husband the whole trip. I hoped that wouldn't become a problem. In any case, we would have to be careful about smoking weed and not get caught.

We usually snowboarded together in a group of four to eight people. None of us were professionals, but we were at least able to master the slopes reasonably safely. Only occasionally did we even dare to ride the black slopes. Only one of us chased down the slopes like a young god: Martin. Watching him could make you a little envious. Sometimes we skied into the forest on the downhill sections and smoked a joint. After that, the boarding feeling intensified considerably. The ski sunglasses conveniently protected us from being unmasked by our red eyes. In the evenings, we drank beer in our rooms or in the disco cellar or went out somewhere in the village to smoke bongs or joints. Of course, there were also some couple stories.

On the third-last day of skiing, we were delighted with the excellent weather. However, it was also quite crowded on the slopes. As usual, we skied in Obertauern. The ski resort had many high-altitude slopes, some even above 2000 meters. The resort was therefore considered snow-sure, even around Easter. But there were always lots of other snow sports enthusiasts out and about. After enjoying our lunch break at an alpine hut with a larger group of people, we took the first descent. I was in a good mood and was skiing fast and taking risks. Suddenly, I lost control due to a small bump that I had seen too late. I tried to regain control by shifting my body weight and changing direction. Suddenly Silke, a girl from our group, was directly in my line of travel and I saw no way of avoiding her. As she didn't make it in time either, we crashed

against each other. I flew forwards and crashed onto my head at high speed. I heard a loud crack somewhere in my cervical spine and ended up lying shocked in the snow.

Suddenly it was very quiet. It seemed like quite a long time; a bit like I was stuck in a time bubble. I must have been doing 60 or 70 kilometers per hour when I crashed; I didn't have time to brake. I felt a bit dizzy, but I wasn't sure if I had hurt myself. The fall had already felt heavy. But after a while I picked myself up and was able to carry on, even though my neck felt funny and was moderately sore. Fortunately, Silke had survived the collision unscathed.

The next day, my neck was stiff. I could hardly move it, and when I did try, there was an unpleasant pain. Well, it must be strained, I thought to myself, and didn't let it spoil my last two days of boarding. A few days earlier, I had already fallen during an unsuccessful jump attempt on a ski jump. Instead of landing on my board, I had crashed onto my left side from a height of three meters and had probably bruised my collarbone; at least that was my assessment. It was swollen and really hurt. Since then, I had avoided all ski jumps. I dampened my accumulated discomfort with a few tablets of ibuprofen. In the evenings, I drank more beer and smoked pot. This made the pain bearable during the last few days of my stay and I was still able to continue boarding.

Back at home, I finally went to my GP as the neck pain still wouldn't go away after a week. He said it was the effects of a whiplash injury, similar to a pulled muscle. After a while, the symptoms would subside on their own.

I could live with that. After a few more days, the neck

pain actually subsided, but didn't disappear completely. Something remained. However, it didn't affect me much at first.

A few weeks later, I went back to my GP because my cervical spine felt dislocated and I had had severe headaches every day for two weeks. He put my cervical spine back into place with a jerky twisting and cracking in both directions and said it should get better in a few days. However, it got worse for a while before it improved again. However, the headaches did not disappear completely, but were still latent.

I didn't think too much about it. At the time, I was just discovering coffee drinking for myself. One cup of coffee in the morning and I was so pumped up that the after-effects of the previous night's bong head were washed away. Even the diffuse headaches were lost in the evening THC rush and the morning coffee rush.

Techno party in Rendsburg

One summer weekend, I went to a techno party near Rendsburg with my school friend Peter and another friend of his. We had a great time together, danced a lot and, to my surprise, I met some friends from Burg. We were relatively far away from home, but as they were also into techno, they had also traveled all the way to the event. The Burg clique was in no way inferior to my clique when it came to smoking weed. I smoked two hash heads with them on a bong in the parking lot. Afterwards, I was so high that I had a panic attack, including a racing heart. I could feel my heart pounding so hard

that I was afraid it might suddenly fail due to overload. I felt so panicked that I was no longer able to talk to anyone. I spent two hours alone in the car until the worst was over.

I was already familiar with conditions like this from smoking weed. It was nothing new. Actually, I almost always developed a certain paranoia, but it was still limited. It mainly occurred because I was afraid of having to deal with adults and parents when I was stoned, because I was hardly in a position to do so. When I had consumed a lot, I found it unpleasant to meet people who hadn't just smoked pot with me and therefore couldn't understand my condition. I then felt stupid because my reaction patterns were slowed down and I was already overwhelmed by normal conversations. This feeling of paranoia was sometimes intensified by a strong feeling of fear, especially when I was high, and sometimes I even had these panic attacks with a racing heart. Fortunately, this happened relatively rarely and I usually put it down to very strong weed or hash. Even though these anxiety and panic attacks didn't leave me feeling good, it was over again after an hour or two and I forgot about it for a while.

However, I noticed that I was increasingly experiencing some of this paranoia and anxiety in my everyday life without being stoned. I observed this with some concern.

Career choice

Many of my peers were starting to think about their career choice. For me, it was still a long way off. I had no concrete idea what profession I wanted to pursue one day. But at least I knew what I didn't

wanted to: To become a farmer and take over my father's farm. As a farmer, you had to work up to 14 hours a day. You didn't get weekends off and no vacation - at least if you kept animals on your farm and didn't have children who could and wanted to take over the work during that time. You had to get up incredibly early, and in winter it was bitterly cold on the farm. You even had to do the work when you were ill.

I wanted to work in the office instead. But I didn't have a plan for what exactly. In the eleventh grade, we had to do a one-week internship, which I completed at a branch of Raiffeisen Bank. But I found it boring. When my mother discovered a job advertisement for a dual study program in the newspaper, she encouraged me to apply for it. You could study business administration at the university of applied sciences in Heide and at the same time do an apprenticeship at the savings bank at the same time. I was already a little interested in business administration, but I couldn't really imagine working at a savings bank. Nevertheless, I applied to see what the application process was like. I was invited to a preliminary test and then to a personal interview in the next round.

Bob Marley Style

I spent a whole afternoon with Falko, who braided and rubbed my dreadlocks for five hours. It really took much longer than I had expected and it was a lot of painstaking manual work. But the result was impressive! As my hair was normally only chin-length, the dreads now hung just above my ears. Some of them had so much tension that they were sticking up wildly in all directions and even at an angle. In any case, they had become quite thick, handsome dreads and I was extremely satisfied. I now had dreadlocks like Bob Marley! How cool was that?

When I came home in the evening, my little seven-year-old brother saw me first. Excited, he ran to our father and shouted: "Dad, Dad, Philip has a spider on his head!".

When my father saw me from his TV chair, he exclaimed in shock: "What do you look like? What have you done to your hair? That looks terrible! I don't want my son walking around like that! You're going to get rid of it!"

I was completely perplexed, because I hadn't expected this reaction at all. My parents were actually quite open to a lot of things. They never really cared about my style of dress, and I was allowed to stay out late in the evenings and go partying if I put in enough effort at school and helped out enough on the farm. I would never have thought that my father would be so bothered by my new hair style.

I replied defiantly: "I'm definitely not going to remove it again! I think it looks very good. It took me five hours to get it like this! After all, it's my look and I have to walk around with it, not you. What do you care? I thought you were a tolerant person!" My father replied in a clearly raised voice: "Have you ever looked in the mirror to see what that looks like? That's not nice at all! You have your interview at the bank in four weeks' time. Are you going to show up like that? I should be ashamed of my son. I don't care if you cut them off or comb them out, but by then these things will be gone!"

I don't give a shit about the interview," I replied. "Do you think I really want to work at the bank?".

Now I was really angry too. I hurriedly stomped up the stairs and slammed the door at the top. 'What's got into him?' I thought. Why is he so upset about my hair? And did he really think I wanted to work at the bank? Did he know me that badly? There was no way I was going to cut off my beautiful new dreads or

to comb it out again. I didn't even know if that would work at all. I would definitely go to the interview like that. After all, it was supposed to be about about my   skills

and not about my clothing style and appearance, right? After a week, I washed my hair for the first time with water and a little curd soap. To my great regret, the dreads came undone. I had thought that if I washed them without shampoo, it wouldn't be a problem, but unfortunately that wasn't the case. The very first time I washed them, they unraveled so much that I had to comb them out and went back to my old hairstyle with chin-length hair. My father didn't say much about it, but I think he was fine with it.

I went to the interview in dress shoes, suit trousers and a light blue T-shirt with the words "Help disabled people". I had an aversion to suits and ties, and since it was a hot day and I didn't want the job anyway, I allowed myself this fun. At the interview, I sat with two other applicants from my class in front of three employees from the savings bank. Unlike me, the other two were of course dressed very neatly. We were each asked to briefly introduce ourselves and then take it in turns to give our opinions on various topics after briefly making up keywords. I was quite nervous in this round. I was so nervous that I didn't put in a good performance. Even when introducing myself, I couldn't really think of what to say apart from my name and age, and I included quite a few "ums". My explanations weren't particularly catchy or comprehensible, and I couldn't present them fluently and confidently either. In the end, my two fellow candidates were both hired and I was turned down. I could only guess whether it was due to my style of dress or my poor performance.

I was a little worried that I had cut such a bad figure in the interview, but that I did not the job didn't make me sad. I was secretly a little proud of my rebellious appearance in the T-shirt. Although, of course, it would have been even more dramatic with dreads!

HASHBROWN COOKIES – A SOLID BUZZ

A different kind of baking mix

I visited my buddy Konstantin at home for the second time. We've been getting on well lately and a special activity was planned for today.

"Come with me, I'll show you something," said Konstantin in a good mood.

"Wow, not bad. Quite big, those plants!" I replied. "When did you harvest them?"

"We cut them off two days ago. They're dry enough by now."

"Cool, the flowers look really fat," I marveled.

Konstantin took a bush from the line on which the plants were hanging to dry and we set about cutting out the flowers. When we had freed all three plants from their flowers, we looked in awe at the large pile that lay before us.

"How many grams of grass do you think that will be?" I asked.

"At least 500 grams," Konstantin estimated. "To be able to bake cookies, we first have to make hemp butter from it".

"Do you know how to make these?"

"Yes, I have a recipe. You boil butter and water together with the hemp in a pot for a few hours and then let it cool down. As the THC is fat-soluble and fat floats to the top, the hemp butter then remains on the surface.

We finally let the whole thing boil for a few hours and squeezed the last bit of liquid butter and hemp mixture out of the hot flowers. It was quite a mess, and it also smelled pretty bad. It then took a few more hours to cool down. All in all, it took almost the whole day until we finally made almost 100 cookies from out of our dough.

In the meantime, Mario, Malte and Freddy had arrived at Konstantin's house. We were sitting at the mixing desk and trying our hand at hip hop trance transitions when Konstantin came in grinning broadly with a full tray of ready-made cookies. I ate three cookies first.

"Mmm ... they even taste really good!"

"Yes, really, I can't wait to see how they hit the spot," said Mario full of anticipation. "I've had hash brown cookies a few times, but will the hemp butter be as good?"

When after 15 minutes there was still no effect, we simply ate a few more cookies. Eventually I had 8 or 9 cookies.

Another ten minutes later, Mario was sitting at the mixing desk when I suddenly noticed how my perception changed. I felt as if my heart started beating to the rhythm of the bass. Half an hour later, I said to the others: "Hey guys, I have to get out of the room!" We left the room and I pulled my baseball cap down over my face because I couldn't stand the brightness any longer. Another hour later, I was all over it. I saw everything as if it was made up of composite honeycombs like a beehive, but also somehow digital, as if I was in a virtual reality simulation. My eyes hurt. It felt like they were about to implode. I decided to take a look in the mirror and winced in horror. The sclera of my eyes, which was normally white, had turned blood red! I looked as if I had just escaped from the chamber of horrors. Driving was out of the question. I was traveling in my parents' second car, which had to be home in the morning. That was an unwritten rule. I had also promised to drive Malte around on the way home. Since driving was out of the question, I decided not to return home until the next morning if I could sober up by then.

The others were also in a good mood by now. Mario and Konstantin had first played soccer outside. In the meantime, however, they had picked up a chainsaw and were playing kung fu with it. They certainly seemed to be having a good time. Freddy had made his way home in good time when he realized that he was getting really wide. My own trip was starting to get really uncomfortable. My heart was racing and panic was setting in.

'I've definitely eaten too many cookies. This must be what it feels like to be on LSD,' I thought. Now I could understand how you can get stuck on a trip. That was way too extreme!

I decided to go to bed and hoped to be back to normal the next morning. But sleeping was out of the question. First my heart started racing and then it stopped for a moment. Shit! I could already see the headline in front of me: "18-year-old suffers heart attack from hash cookies". I also had the uneasy feeling that if I did survive, my condition could stay that way. Perhaps my brain had simply been overloaded by too many impressions, emotions and thoughts? Just burnt out? It was a horror trip. I desperately wanted to be normal again - not some kind of stuck freak who can no longer use his brain properly. Thoughts like that flashed through my mind. But after an hour or two in panic mode, I must have fallen asleep after all.

I woke up around nine o'clock and was relieved to find that I was somewhat recovered. I still felt a certain distortion of perception, but it was nothing compared to last night. However, I was slightly worried that this extreme experience might have permanently damaged some of my synapses.

When I arrived home at 11 a.m., my parents gave me a hell of a time because I didn't bring the car back until now - and also because I didn't let them know.

I ignored it as best I could. Afterwards, I went back to bed with a guilty conscience because I was still too exhausted to cope with the world.

My relationship with my parents had been deteriorating for a few years now, ever since I started partying, drinking and smoking weed. I spent less and less time at home and more and more time out with friends.

In addition, I didn't like talking to my parents when I was stoned. And since I was relatively often stoned, I reduced communication to a minimum at such times and avoided them. Since I had increasingly persistent and severe headaches and neck pain, I was also often extremely irritable, grumpy and depressed.

My father kept trying to have a normal conversation with me. But I often reacted irritably and choked off the conversation. In hindsight, I often felt sorry for this, but I couldn't help it in the situation. There was a constant tension in the air that was difficult to bear for everyone involved. Occasionally, this tension erupted into conflicts and arguments. My mother in particular could sometimes say mean and hurtful things when she got very angry. This would hurt me and I would retaliate as best I could with nasty, verbal retaliation. As I discovered, I wasn't so bad at saying mean things either!

BEFORE GRADUATION - THE CREEPING DECLINE

The last school year

At the beginning of year 13, the difficulties really started. I felt exhausted in the morning and my eyes were completely swollen shut every morning. I also had a slight pressure in my head, in the front of my temples to be precise. 'It's probably my eyes from smoking so much weed', I thought, 'chronically broken from overstimulation'. I was able to wash away the pressure in my head with strong coffee in the morning, and it usually disappeared during the day so that I didn't feel it anymore in the afternoon. Unfortunately, it was always there again the next morning.

I also noticed that I occasionally fell into low moods. If I had smoked a lot the night before, I was still a bit apathetic the next morning. Some days I even found it difficult to talk to anyone at all because I didn't really know what to talk about. My head just didn't want to spit out anything meaningful. During the breaks, I didn't really know what to do with myself. It was downright exhausting to have conversations with friends and classmates. I withdrew more and more, and on the worse days I tried to make myself invisible. This went on for quite some time. The pressure in my temples got a little stronger and stayed a little longer, well into the late afternoon.

Despite everything, I still managed to pass my A-levels quite well, with a final grade of 2.5. I had just pulled myself together in the two years of upper school, did my homework regularly again, studied for exams and even made an effort to participate orally in lessons as much as possible. Nevertheless, I didn't limit myself too much in terms of parties and friends. My parents had always said: "If you can party, you can get up early and work." Although these sayings always annoyed me, they were somehow programmed into me. In addition to all the partying, it had always been important to me to get good grades in order to maintain my chances of getting into a good university. After all, our school was known for having a certain standard. I was happy with the result.

Unsuccessful treatment attempts

The pressure in my head increased slowly but steadily. When a permanent pain also settled in my neck, I began to take the matter a little more seriously. So I went to an orthopaedist for the first time. He examined me by carrying out various mobility tests on my neck and arms and asking me a few questions about the pain. He then prescribed me six sessions of physiotherapy. The prescription said "cervical spine syndrome, cervical syndrome". This was probably a fairly general diagnosis that meant that you had complaints in the neck or shoulder area. I was first shown some exercises to strengthen my back muscles. At the fourth or fifth appointment, the physiotherapist tried to mobilize my neck area. She massaged and stretched the neck area.

I thought that was so bad that I exclaimed in horror: "Aaahhh!!! ... That's very painful! Are you sure you're doing the right thing?"

"The muscles are very hard and tense. That can sometimes cause pain. You have to get through it!" the physiotherapist assured me confidently.

After the treatment I was shocked at the pain I had to endure. I had been on the verge of tears several times. But I hoped that the treatment would soon have a positive effect. But even after the treatment, my neck still hurt really badly. For two weeks, this pain in my neck, which had been greatly intensified by the treatment, was a constant companion. I moaned the whole time, was extremely irritable and cursed the physiotherapist. I skipped the last two appointments. I didn't want to put myself through this ordeal again.

The next time I went to the orthopaedist, he prescribed me a TENS unit instead. It was supposed to reduce the perception of pain through electrical stimulation. You stuck the four small electrode pads on the neck area and could then use the device to regulate the intensity of the electric shocks. When the intensity was set to maximum, the muscles began to twitch. It even felt reasonably pleasant and I used the device once or several times a day for a few weeks. But I couldn't see any positive effect. After these futile attempts, I decided to try again with another orthopaedist.

In the meantime, I also noticed a certain anxiety in me. I was no longer as quick-witted in conversations as I had been in previous years. It was also more difficult to speak. Social situations were now more stressful for me as they were always disturbed by a slight pain. In close circles of friends, where we were familiar with each other, it still went quite well. But it was with people I didn't know so well that interaction became increasingly difficult. So I began to avoid such situations.

CIVILIAN SERVICE - IT'S A PAIN IN THE NECK

Civilian life

As I found it difficult to imagine carrying a weapon and the strict regiment of the German army, I decided against it early on and opted for civilian service. I liked the idea of doing social work for other people. I was also toying with the idea of studying social education after my civilian service. So I applied for a community service position in outpatient nursing and care at the German Red Cross.

My tasks included washing a bedridden old man in the morning and changing the bed linen. This task took a lot of effort at first, but became easier over time. I found that I got used to a lot of things. I had my own car from the DRK, which I used to drive from patient to patient throughout the district. I looked after some patients, who I pushed around the villages in a wheelchair, ran errands for them and accompanied elderly ladies to the hairdresser. I also had a blind patient with whom I went on a tandem bike ride once a week. Despite the increasing restrictions due to the pain in my head and neck, I was still on top form at parties. I had been dating Annika from Brunsbüttel since the summer. We had met on a ski trip and met again at a few parties. I was totally smitten. We went to open airs and discos together, went on vacation together and experienced many wonderful moments.

The problem with the pressure in my head got worse and worse during this time. The pain continued to increase and eventually did not disappear during the course of the day.

Then there was also the increasing pain in my neck. My attention and mood suffered as a result.

Tension in the neck, tension at home

I continued to live at home. However, I got on worse and worse with my parents. When I wasn't spending time with Annika, I was usually working a part-time job as a pizza driver or visiting friends at home, where we usually indulged in our favorite hobby - smoking weed. However, I realized that I wasn't tolerating it so well anymore. Even when I was high, I couldn't think of any funny anecdotes, and my linguistic skills deteriorated even more.

Overall, I had the feeling that things were going downhill all round. I tried to avoid my parents completely when I was stoned. And when I wasn't stoned, I was irritable because of the constant headaches and neck pain. I hardly talked to them anymore. What was I supposed to talk to them about? We lived in such different worlds! I especially didn't feel like talking to my father. He made an effort and often tried to start a conversation with me. But I couldn't get a flowing conversation going because I had a headache and it took too much energy to put my thoughts into words. The tension in my neck usually became more uncomfortable and the headache worse just when he wanted to talk to me. I hated this feeling and got angry with my father because he wanted to talk to me right now and was making my pain worse. At the same time, I was also angry with myself because I was incapable of having a sensible conversation with my father. He didn't deserve that!

I began to hate the tension in my neck, the pressure and pain in my left and right temples to hate this permanently restricted state. They made my life hell and I could no longer behave like a reasonable person. That's why I usually reacted dismissively and irritably. This behavior eventually led to us almost only talking to each other when my parents complained or were angry with me. I developed a real dislike of them, because all I got from them was arguments and anger. I no longer liked being at home and when I was there, I just watched TV.

Everyday combat zone

I had actually expected that it would make me feel good to help other people. And it was also the case that the patients were usually happy when I came to see them. It was often the highlight of their week, or so it seemed to me. But I didn't get so many positive things out of it myself. Because everything was becoming more and more stressful for me, I was particularly aware of the suffering, illnesses and loneliness of the elderly. That dragged me down even further rather than giving me any satisfaction from helping. By now, every day was a struggle. I was constantly in a bad mood and began to see many things in a negative light. Even in my relationship with Annika, I only saw the unpleasant things. As a result, my constant irritability only got worse when we were together. I could no longer enjoy our togetherness and felt less and less that I loved her. Maybe we weren't compatible? Maybe it had something to do with my fundamental dissatisfaction? I didn't know, but I didn't see a future for us either. So I broke up with my girlfriend, who I had been with for six months, just before Christmas.

My civilian service lasted a total of 13 months, and the first half was now over. I was now enjoying the work no longer at all. I could only bear the suffering of these people with difficulty, because I already had enough to do with my own suffering. My headaches and neck pain got worse from day to day and slowly became really dramatic. Especially all the wheelchair pushing in Burg was poison for my neck, because it was quite hilly there. The lady I was pushing around there wasn't exactly a beanpole either. In the evening, I tried to relax my battered neck with a neck pillow, which I warmed up in the microwave. The warmth felt good for a short time, but it hardly helped with the pain.

Normal painkillers only had a minor effect. I hardly noticed anything from a standard 400 ibuprofen tablet. If I took two of them, I was able to reduce the pain by 20 to 30 percent for a while. I experimented a few times with over-the-counter painkillers, but on the whole I took them sporadically as the pain-relieving effect was simply too small.

Due to the constant pain, my mood got worse and worse. Sometimes I wondered whether a psychiatrist would classify this condition as depressive. Especially when I was stoned, the tension and pain made it so difficult for me to express myself that I often felt quite stupid. I couldn't see through a lot of things so quickly either. For example, when the rules for a new card or board game were explained to a group of friends, I had enormous problems remembering them and understanding the game. I had to keep asking for the rules and made lots of little mistakes. I noticed that my friends found it much easier.

It was clear: my cognitive abilities were on the decline.

There were still a few bright moments when I drank a lot of alcohol at parties at the weekend. The alcohol numbed the pain and loosened up my muscles and I was able to articulate myself much better. However, I could no longer chat people up like I used to. The infamous Philip jokes that I used to conjure up from my creative bag of tricks were now just a memory. The well had dried up.

Physician frustration and neck stretching

During my community service, I was treated by a new orthopaedic surgeon. I was very hopeful that he would finally help me. On my first visit, the doctor gave me a local anesthetic injection in my neck. The pain was a little more bearable for a few days afterwards, but then the effect wore off pretty quickly.

He had also recommended that I do regular strength training or go swimming. I then bought a card for the gym in Meldorf. I worked out there once or twice a week and went to the sauna. The warmth of the sauna did have a relaxing effect. However, as the situation hadn't really improved after a few weeks, but rather got worse, I made another appointment with the orthopaedist. He fired the second salvo from the catalog of measures. Every time I went to the doctor, they put me in an apparatus that was supposed to stretch my neck. It looked a bit like an instrument of torture, but fortunately it didn't hurt, it was just a bit uncomfortable. The doctor also prescribed me a referral for an MRI scan and tetrazepam tablets to relax my muscles. Stretching my neck didn't have any noticeable effect. The MRI scan was also inconclusive. There were no abnormal findings: there was no physical damage to the cervical spine.

However, the tetrazepam tablets really hit the spot. One

tablet made the muscles in my entire body go limp, so that I was extremely relaxed. The headaches and neck pain also disappeared almost completely for a few hours. When I took a tablet like this, I was able to function fairly normally again. I was also able to speak and formulate to some extent again. However, I also felt a bit like I was on a drug. I was actually supposed to take the tablets at night, but that didn't have much effect. I preferred to take them during the day instead. However, I shouldn't take them every day as they had addictive potential. In addition, the effect diminished considerably if you took a tablet several days in a row. So I saved the tablets for special occasions when I wanted to be in a good mood or had to function well - or for days when the pain was so bad that I couldn't bear it at all.

My last visit to the orthopaedist was two weeks before the end of my community service. I asked him to put me on sick leave for the next two weeks due to chronic tension headaches, as I no longer felt able to cope with my everyday working life.

In addition to the sick note, he also gave me a tip for the future: "If you're studying in Kiel, go and have a few beers with your colleagues. Alcohol relaxes the muscles."

That was all he had to offer? I thought it was inappropriate for such advice to come from a doctor. He was now the third doctor I had consulted about my complaints and the results were frustrating. More than two years had now passed since my snowboarding accident and I had sought help from the very beginning. But despite the various therapy measures, it only got worse instead of better.

Self-diagnosis

After this experience, I made a decision: If this kind of advice was the best help I could expect from a doctor, then perhaps I'd better look for therapy measures that worked myself. In the second half of my community service, I had already started to deal with my illness more intensively. I searched the internet for information on the terms chronic pain, tension headaches, depression, migraine, neck pain, whiplash.

My self-diagnosis was: Chronic tension headache with neck tension, probably with a little depressive mood on top. I had read somewhere on the internet that more than ten percent of all whiplash patients develop chronic tension headaches. My theory was that a whole series of negative factors came together in my case. As a teenager, I had suffered from back pain for a while and had undergone physiotherapy for

I got a "hunched back". My back posture really wasn't the best. The key event was the snowboarding accident with the whiplash injury. Other factors were the frequent smoking weed and drinking alcohol, as well as the permanently poor relationship with my parents. Perhaps my severe heartbreak, which I had suffered at the age of sixteen, also played a role. I also had a hunch that the one or other horror trip and the panic attacks I sometimes had from smoking weed contributed to it. So I put my clinical picture together like a complicated puzzle.

I had read that if the headache occurred more than 20 days a month, it could be described as chronic. That was the case for me, because I now had it every day - from the moment I woke up in the morning to the moment I went to sleep at night.

The process of pain chronification has been described on the Internet described in more detail. If pain occurs permanently over a long period of time, a so-called pain memory is formed. This means that the neurotransmitter constellation that generates the pain signal occurs even if there is no longer any underlying physical cause of the pain. If the process has already progressed so far that an intensive pain memory has formed, this is a disease in itself. It can reinforce itself in a vicious circle. Due to the constant pain, the body produces fewer endorphins and neurotransmitters, which normally have a pain-relieving effect. The result is that the pain is perceived even more intensely. This in turn means that even fewer endorphins are produced and the pain seems stronger. The pain signal "burns" itself deep into the nerve pathways.

Various therapeutic measures were mentioned in my online sources: Physiotherapy, local anesthetic injections, progressive muscle relaxation, autogenic training, biofeedback, acupuncture, acupressure, yoga, meditation, pain-inhibiting tricyclic antidepressants and, last but not least, opiates for particularly bad cases.

What should I study?

I decided to look for a new doctor as soon as I started studying. It wouldn't be long until then.

Before that, I had something else important to clarify. In the meantime, I had given up on studying something social. I simply didn't enjoy my everyday community service enough and it had put me off. But I definitely knew that I wanted to study. I didn't want to work eight hours a day and wanted to put it off for as long as possible.

Now that I had ruled out social pedagogy, I was interested in psychology, sociology and business administration. I received more information about the content and access to the course at a student advisory service at the careers information center. Psychology was a highly sought-after subject and the numerus clausus was

1.2, so it was out of the question as I had an average grade of 2.5. I also didn't feel able to treat other people in my current condition. Sociology sounded exciting in terms of content, but what could you become with it? I kept hearing the saying that sociologists later drove cabs. When the consultant also mentioned that she had studied sociology, I decided on business studies. That was a safe bet. After graduating, you still had the opportunity to develop in different sectors and directions. It wouldn't be too difficult for me to find a job, I told myself. My parents would certainly welcome this choice too: business studies wasn't too intellectual, but reasonably down-to-earth. I also had a good feel for money and entrepreneurship. The subject would suit me, I was sure of that.

In my current condition, however, I couldn't work because of the pain. I took sick leave for the last two weeks of my community service because of the headaches, as I didn't feel able to cope with the work. I hoped that this would improve again when my life situation changed.

Introduction to meditation at the adult education center

There weren't many mental challenges during my civilian service. I spent a lot of time with older people who told me the same stories over and over again. They were often war stories. My part-time job as a pizza delivery boy wasn't necessarily a challenge either.

I therefore decided to continue my education at the adult education center so that the start of my studies would not be quite so difficult. I got hold of a course program and chose a Spanish beginners' course in Meldorf. I wanted to learn something new, but also something useful. Spanish appealed to me because there were many countries where it was spoken.

I also read the chapters on health and relaxation with interest. There were courses in healthy eating, back training, tai chi, yoga and introduction to meditation. I was particularly interested in the latter course. Perhaps it could help me with my complaints?

I asked my friend Ralle if he wanted to come along. I didn't have to persuade him for long because Ralle was always pretty open to new things. I used to play basketball with him at the club. He was also interested in computers, was generally a keen sportsman and liked to party. So we had quite a lot in common and I was pleased that he wanted to come with me.

The course consisted of eight evenings, each lasting an hour and a half, at the adult education center in Heide. On the first evening of the course, we all gathered in a medium-sized meeting room. With his calm charisma, the course leader immediately struck me as very likeable. I noticed with unease that a former teacher of mine was also among the participants. We were a group of eight people, young and old, a colorful mix. The course leader introduced himself and told us that he had been traveling to India frequently for many years to practice yoga and meditation. He then asked us for a short round of introductions. We were also asked to explain why we were interested in meditation and what we hoped to gain from the course.

I immediately noticed how my pre-existing excitement and anxiety grew into nervous fear. There was no way I wanted to be in front of my buddy and had to admit to my former teacher that I was suffering from chronic pain, that it had possibly developed into depression and that I was now hoping that meditation would help me. That would be embarrassing! But what should I say instead? I noticed how my neck muscles tensed up and the pressure in my head increased. This always happened in awkward situations now.

I could no longer think properly at all. Now I was worried whether I would be able to get any words out at all in this state. Panic! My heart was pounding like crazy. I wondered if the others could see how fast my heart was beating. 'It's best if I lean forward a little so that my T-shirt isn't so tight against my body,' I thought. 'Do I have a red head? Shit, what am I supposed to say now?

Fifty percent of my attention was focused on the panic and 30 percent on the pain in my neck. The remaining 20 percent were feverishly trying to come up with a few sentences. Two more participants, then it was my turn. I didn't hear what the others were saying; I was too preoccupied with myself.

'How can that be?' I asked myself. 'It's just a harmless little round of introductions! You briefly say who you are and what you want here, and that's it! No big deal! Why are you so scared of it? There's no logical reason for it. Philip, you need to calm down now!'

When it was finally my turn, I managed to squeeze out a few shaky sentences: "I'm Philip, I'm currently doing my community service with the German Red Cross and I'm 19 years old. And why I'm interested in meditation, um ... I'm just curious."

Once I had said that, a huge weight was lifted off my shoulders and I calmed down a bit. Man, it would have been embarrassing if I hadn't said a word in front of my buddy and a former teacher! What would they have thought of me? I'm sure they would have thought I was a bit mentally unwell. That probably wasn't
so far from the truth. But I couldn't imagine that it would be a good idea to let my buddies know. They would probably start avoiding me.

As the evening progressed, we did various small perception and concentration exercises. This was also the case in the later sessions. At one point, we were asked to gaze into a candle in the middle of our circle of chairs for five minutes. Then we were asked to repeat a mantra or pay attention to our breathing for a few minutes. After each exercise, there was another round in which everyone was asked to share their experiences. In these rounds, too, the feeling of tension increased again and the anxiety came up. However, it wasn't quite as paralyzing and panicky as in the first round. This time, you didn't really have to say anything about yourself.

Although I found the exercises interesting, the discussion groups really got to me, so I always went to these evenings with extremely mixed feelings. By the end of the course, I had gained an insight into various meditation techniques and yoga, but I couldn't really apply them on this basis. That disappointed me a little, because I would have liked to go deeper.

The low point

On a warm Saturday evening in summer, I was walking along the flagstone path near our house. The sun was shining and still had power. I could hear the buzzing sound of crickets and was surrounded by idyllic nature. To my right was the Klevhang, the former cliff. To my left was the expanse of the marshland, where I could see as far as the next dyke. The flagstone path led along the Klevhang, which at that time separated the sea from the land and today separates the marsh from the Geest landscape.

However, I wasn't in the mood to enjoy it all. I was usually out with friends on Saturday nights - at discos, open-air festivals or just drinking and smoking weed at someone's house. But over the last few months and weeks, my headaches and neck pain had become increasingly unbearable. Most of the time, I no longer enjoyed spending time with friends. I found it hard to concentrate on conversations and usually didn't have much to say. This frustrated me as I could no longer score points with my wit and humor - as if I was suddenly someone else. I only reacted, if at all, and no longer acted. That made me feel inferior.

As I went for a walk, I thought about my decision to stay at home that evening. I thought about the last few weeks and months, and also about the future. On the one hand, I was glad that I had stayed at home again today. Anything else would have been torture. On the other hand, I was worried that this was slowly distancing me from my friends and that I would become increasingly lonely if something didn't fundamentally change about my condition.

I could clearly feel the pressure in my head, especially at my temples. This pressure was extremely uncomfortable and took up so much of my attention that I couldn't think clearly. When the pressure was as strong as it was today, I could only speak simple sentences, had to think a lot and spoke uncertainly and somewhat confusedly. In such a state, I couldn't impress anyone, make anyone laugh or convince anyone of anything. Then I was a heap of misery.

When I felt the pressure, I could feel it particularly on the top half of my head. It surrounded my head like an invisible helmet. However, the worst part was in the back of my neck, in the upper part of the cervical spine. Everything started from there. That was the origin.

I couldn't hold my attention for too long because it caused so much aversion and pain. I could no longer turn my head all the way to the left and right. The freedom of movement was restricted and the turning itself was so uncomfortable that I tried to do it as rarely as possible.

The pain and the restrictions that came with it were so frustrating and grueling that I had a bleak outlook for my future. After the snowboarding accident, I had had a year of discomfort, which was still quite bearable. But in the last year, the pain, anxiety and speech problems had increased more and more. I no longer felt like meeting up with friends in this state. How could I manage to study? How was I supposed to find work later on? How was I supposed to find new friends, let alone a new girlfriend? How could I lead a happy, fulfilled life in this state?

None of this was conceivable with this pain. I couldn't even have a normal conversation anymore. All the visits to orthopaedists and physiotherapists had so far brought no improvement at all. On the contrary, all my efforts had been in vain and things were going from bad to worse. So far, no one had been able to help me and I couldn't see any way out of this misery. I was also pretty sure that I was now depressed - although I couldn't really assess how bad it was.

I was deeply ashamed of it and didn't talk about it with my parents, friends or doctors. I thought that if I started talking about it, I would also have to talk about my marijuana and hashish use. Then everyone would immediately conclude that it was all down to that. Then I would immediately be labeled a "druggie" and maybe even to be labeled a "psycho". I definitely didn't want that! It wasn't that simple. And I didn't believe that psychotherapy or psychotropic drugs would help me either.

For me, the root of all evil was the fall and snowboarding accident and the pain in my neck, which then led to other psychological problems. And then everything spiraled upwards in a self-reinforcing vicious circle.

I felt overwhelmed by hopelessness - and thought about whether it would be better to end my life. Was that the best way to stop feeling all the suffering? Maybe that would also spare my family the misery that dealing with me had become and would possibly become. After all, I was just irritable, bad-tempered and taciturn. Almost every conversation with my parents ended in an argument.

However, I didn't know what came after death. Was it all just over then, or did it continue somehow? It seemed more likely to me that it continued, in whatever way. Maybe rebirth and karma really did exist. It still seemed exotic to me. But somehow I had the feeling that suicide was not the solution. Because of this feeling, I decided that suicide was out of the question for me. I had to look for other ways to get out of this bad situation.

SIDDHARTA - ON THE TRAIL OF POVERTY, KARMA AND THE DALAI LAMA

The magic of Siddharta

When I was 18, I came across the book Siddhartha by Hermann Hesse. Written in beautiful language, I practically devoured it. It was about a young, handsome, wealthy Brahmin who lived in India at the time of the Buddha and decided to go on a spiritual quest. As a young man, he left home and spent several years in the forest practicing meditation and asceticism. After a few years, however, he ended his asceticism. He had learned tremendous spiritual discipline. But he had the feeling that this could not be everything and that there had to be more.

He then also met the Buddha. He was deeply impressed by the Buddha's charisma, but refused to join him. He wanted to find his own path. Instead, he turned to the worldly life, learned the art of the Kama Sutra with a playmate, became a wealthy merchant thanks to his skills and took a liking to wine and gambling. More and more his spiritual discipline dried up and he became more and more of an ordinary person who became entangled in worldly life.

At an advanced age, he realized that this way of life was also making him increasingly dissatisfied, and he turned his back on this life too. He went to an old ferryman who had once ferried him across the river and whose calm charisma had remained in his memory. From then on, he lived the quiet life of a ferryman, meditated by the river and finally attained enlightenment at the end of his life.

This book cast a magical spell over me. I felt the desire, just like the young Brahmin, to discover the secrets of consciousness and learn how the mind worked. I felt this would be a worthwhile pursuit in life. Besides, I could imagine that it might help me with the pain. The best thing to do, I thought, would be to become a meditation teacher. Then I would also have a good motivation to explore the mind more and more deeply, as I would be obliged to give good instructions to my students.

I wondered whether I could do it professionally and make a living from it. Meditation was not a recognized profession in our society and the image was more esoteric. To really be able to function as a recognized meditation teacher, I would have to meditate for several years in a cave and in isolation. There I would have to gain the necessary experience and skills to gain really deep insights and be taken seriously. At least that was my impression after reading the book. I couldn't see any other way for me. After all, there was no university where you could study this. Besides, everyone I knew would more or less ridicule me as an esoteric crank.

As I didn't want to leave everything behind and couldn't imagine spending the next few years in a cave, I left my plan to study business administration. Perhaps at some point in my life I would have the opportunity to do more meditation. I discarded this fantastic thought experiment for the time being and applied for a place at university in Kiel.

I also wanted to go to India and see this exotic, wild country. I had been toying with the idea of traveling there for some time. But ever since I read Siddhartha, I was magically drawn there. The people there believed in many different gods and in reincarnation. There were also many gurus, yoga and the Buddha, who all had a connection with this country.

There was poverty and modern software companies, sacred cows and hippies in Goa. Although I was already struggling to cope with my everyday life in Germany, it tempted me and sounded like a breathtaking adventure.

I had saved up quite a bit in the previous year. By delivering pizzas, occasionally driving my father's tractor and doing community service with the German Red Cross, I had managed to put 3000 marks on the high side. I had developed an interest in shares through a stock market game at school. My mother had also recently opened a share portfolio and subscribed to Telekom shares when they went public. I followed my intuition that share trading was a trend with potential and opened a securities account at my savings bank. While I was still doing my civilian service, I invested 2000 marks in Telekom shares and 1000 marks in a Internet investment fund. Six months later, the stock market boom had doubled the value to 6,000 marks. By the end of my civilian service, I had a bulging travel fund to travel around India for seven weeks until my studies began. Many of my friends also wanted to travel to India, but unfortunately none of them had the money. So I set off on my own - and flew to New Delhi.

Arrival in India

I looked out of the window at the buildings on the airport grounds as our plane landed in New Delhi. The buildings looked strange; not like buildings normally look, but somehow surreal. They didn't look modern or old, and their purpose was difficult to discern. I began to suspect that I had really arrived in a completely different world.

India! What on earth had possessed me to come here, all by myself? The Goa parties I had visited in recent years? The mixture of psychedelic trance music, Indian flair with scarves, incense sticks, black light, chai tea and the smell of grass had always made a big impression on me. It was definitely also the book about Siddhartha Gautama by Hermann Hesse. Or maybe it was the religious education lessons at school where we studied Hinduism? At the time, I couldn't understand how such a crazy religion with thousands of gods could exist. But that's exactly what made it so fascinating.

I was on the run and also on the search. I was fleeing from the pain and the miserable everyday life that resulted from it, and I was looking for a better way of being. All I knew was that everything in my life was shit at the time and I saw no way out. However, I also knew that I was fascinated by topics such as meditation, Hinduism, Buddhism and yoga - perhaps because they seemed so exotic and difficult to grasp. But certainly also because I was hoping for a solution to my problems.

My initial unease in this strange, new world was mitigated by the fact that the border official who checked my passport was extremely friendly. "Is this your first time in India?" he asked, smiling at me with a broad smile.

"Uh, yeah, my first time."

"Then have a nice trip!" he replied, smiling even more broadly. It was a thoroughly sincere smile, the kind you rarely get from strangers in Germany. And I had certainly never met such friendly border officials in Germany ... At a bank counter in the reception hall, I changed 100 marks into around 2000 rupees, left the airport building and boarded a bus heading towards the city center.

On the way towards the center, I saw poverty on a large scale right before my eyes for the first time in my life. Many of the houses looked like small Wooden shacks. People were sitting, standing and loitering everywhere. I wondered what this or that person was doing at the moment and whether they had been sitting by the side of the road all day. The traffic roared loudly, the air was stuffy from the dust and exhaust fumes, and yet there were mothers with their small children sitting right on the central reservation. Some were begging, others were vegetating there, and from time to time I also saw some lifeless bodies lying there, or so it seemed to me. This extreme confrontation with poverty, suffering, dirt and noise overwhelmed me. I clearly had a huge culture shock.

This was only going to get worse. As I didn't know where the bus was going and none of the passengers spoke English, I was dropped off at a place that at least somewhat resembled a city center. However, it couldn't be compared to any city center I knew. There were no Mac Donalds, skyscrapers or modern office buildings anywhere. Instead, it was full of shacks, poor people and traffic. There I was with my backpack, 20 years young, all alone in the middle of New Delhi and without a clue where I actually was.

The temperature was over 40 degrees and all the poor people frightened me. At the same time, I felt enormous compassion for them. I had seen slums and poverty on TV, but it was a completely different dimension to be in the middle of it all at once. As soon as I got off the bus, a friendly Indian man came up to me and wanted to talk to me, show me all sorts of things - and sell me a watch. Although he was friendly, I felt suspicious and after what seemed like an eternity, I finally shook him off. Then a rickshaw driver started to work me over until I finally got in and let him drive me to a budget hotel that I had picked out of the Lonely Planet.

Unfortunately, the hotel did not turn out to be a stroke of luck. My room was totally run down. There was a noisy building site in front of the hotel and the ceiling fan was hanging at an angle from the ceiling.

You had to be afraid of being hit by it at night. It also only ran at a snail's pace, which was quite an ordeal given the temperatures. I slept very little that night and dozed off somewhere between panic and culture shock. If my return flight hadn't been booked in seven weeks' time, I would have preferred to fly back the very next day. But that wasn't possible - at least I wouldn't have known how. Besides, it would have been pretty embarrassing to give up so quickly.

After a hot night without much rest, I made my way back to the city on foot with my backpacker's rucksack on my back. The thermometer was already over 40 degrees again in the morning and I was sweating even when I was sitting down. However, the enormous heat had a strange effect on my neck muscles. After two days in the heat, they relaxed so much that my neck no longer hurt. I could even move my head better to the left and right again. What's more, my headaches, which had been a permanent feature of my life for a long time, suddenly disappeared almost completely. I also noticed that it was easier for me to speak again, even in English. Without the pain in my frontal temporal lobe, it seemed to take me less energy to turn thoughts into words.

I was all alone in Delhi, had a culture shock, was tired and physically weak from the heat - but I felt happier than I had for a long time. I was pain-free. I could move my neck. I saw light at the end of the tunnel again. Now everything would get better!

Indian Switzerland

However, my euphoria at being pain-free only lasted a few days. I booked a bus trip to Kashmir, a high plateau at an altitude of 2000 meters in the Himalayas. It was only 25 degrees there, and my neck pain and headaches soon returned in their usual way. For a few days, I lived on a houseboat on Lake Srinagar. Two employees cooked for me and accompanied me when I wanted to see the place. Together with the employees, I also smoked black hash and watched the German crime series Derrick in black and white in English. I found that quite funny, as the English dubbing seemed extremely amateurish to me.

Marijuana grew on every street corner, and smoking tobacco, marijuana and hashish seemed to be widespread and socially acceptable here. Men with water pipes could be seen everywhere. There were so-called floating fields on Lake Srinagar, which were cultivated by sun-tanned men. Often these workers even had a large water pipe in their boats, which they puffed on with relish while working.

After I had spent a good week in Kashmir, one of the houseboat employees got me a bus ticket and put me on the bus to Jammu in the morning. We spent the whole day on the bus, driving up and down hills through the breathtaking mountain landscape The buses in India were just as colorful as the women's colorful saris. There were red, yellow or blue buses, mostly with abstract decorations and paintings. There was a large jukebox next to the driver, from which Hindi music was constantly blaring so loudly that you could hardly have a conversation with the person sitting next to you. I enjoyed driving through the untouched nature of the mountains to this exotic music. A pleasant breeze blew in through the open windows, along with a little dust here and there.

On the edge of the Himalayas

My stomach had been in turmoil since the second day in India and my digestive mode alternated between constipation and diarrhea. As my stomach often grumbled and gurgled and sometimes hurt, I only bought cookies during our stops and made do with that. Although the day was slowly coming to an end, the unfamiliar and oppressive heat of the city almost killed me when we arrived in Jammu. The hot air seemed to be literally building up in front of the mountains. Jammu made a very crowded, noisy and dusty impression on me. So far, I hadn't seen a single tourist or person from the West. Even in the Lonely Planet, which I had studied extensively during the bus ride, there were only a few entries about Jammu.

To my delight, I found out that the home of the Dalai Lama and the Tibetans in exile was not far away. Of course I had heard of the Dalai Lama before, but I didn't know that he lived in India with many other Tibetans. I thought it was actually quite nice of the Indians to take in so many Tibetan refugees. I really wanted to see this and travel on there straight away.

As we only reached Jammu late in the evening, there was no possibility of taking another connecting bus. So I had to stay in Jammu for one night. I asked a few hotels directly at the bus station for accommodation and had them show me the rooms. As they all looked very run-down and unhygienic, I finally decided to stay in one of the shabby rooms anyway due to a lack of alternatives. I paid 120 rupees for one night including dinner. That was the equivalent of about 3 marks.

We ate rice with dal, which I ate somewhat skeptically. I was joined by one of the hotel employees and we got chatting. I had noticed that there were many holy men here with long hair and orange robes, so-called sadhus.

They renounced worldly life and wandered through India as dispossessed holy men. I asked the man: "There are so many sadhus here. Are they really all real holy men?"

He replied: "Oh, many of them are drug addicts, some are even dangerous. But there are also some who are truly honorable holy men in search of their God. Some even have supernatural abilities and can, for example, materialize objects from dust or stones. I have witnessed this myself with my own eyes."

When I inspected my room a little more closely, I noticed that there was a very unpleasant smell coming from the bathroom.

"This place has probably never been cleaned with detergent," I thought. Between my legs, two big fat cockroaches scurried out of the bathroom and into my bedroom, and I almost went into cardiac arrest. Large insects had always frightened and disgusted me. The cockroaches eventually disappeared into some hole and I stretched my mosquito net over the filthy mattress. I put my sleeping bag on the mattress so that I didn't have to touch it when I slept; it would surely be swarming with bugs. Now the mosquitoes were slowly coming in through the open window. I started to feel slightly paranoid because of all the insects. 'They must have malaria here if it's always this hot,' I thought and curled up on the bed so that I wasn't touching the mosquito net on either side. I didn't want to give either the cockroaches or the mosquitoes anything to attack.

I hardly slept a wink all night and left the hotel just after sunrise at four in the morning. I had never stayed in such a dump before. I decided to choose my rooms better in future and not to be too stingy with the accommodation costs - even though there were no better options here anyway.

In Dharamsala, the home of the Dalai Lama

The bus to my destination left at seven in the morning, and again I spent almost a whole day on the road. It took a long time for the old bus to work its way up the 1500 meters of altitude at which Dharamsala lay. The climate here was completely different to that in Jammu. It was damp and clammy, and occasionally we sank into the clouds. The houses and people also looked very different to what I had seen in India before.

After sleeping in the next day, I treated myself to a really good breakfast of toast and cheese, jam and Nescafé. It was pretty much the best coffee you could get. India, as I had come to know it so far, was a country of tea and not a country of coffee. You could get chai tea on every corner and on every occasion. But for me as a coffee junkie, the coffee was usually not a real treat.

After breakfast, I went for a walk and had a look around the town. It was a manageable size. Everything here looked very different from the rest of India. The houses were more solidly built, everything was quite clean and orderly. Most people had the typical narrow eyes and roundish facial features associated with Tibetans. I saw some monks who were dressed in brown robes and had no hair on their heads.

There were also many white tourists from different countries. Because of the tourists, there were also more western products to buy here. There were even restaurants serving pizza and pasta. Although we were high up in the mountains, there were also internet cafés and telephone stores where you could make overseas calls. This western cultural influence actually made me feel a little more at home in this foreign world.

I noticed many bookshops were in addition to the typical

travel guides and novels, there was a large selection of books on Tibetan Buddhism, as well as life guides and books on spiritual topics. Other stores sold energetic healing stones and offered special acupressure and energy massages. This place consisted of an exotic little world of Buddhism and attracted spiritual seekers from all over the world. This mixture also had a certain attraction for me.

I noticed a small store with a sign saying "Reiki healing", which aroused my curiosity. I plucked up my courage and asked the young Indian man sitting in the store what Reiki was. He was very friendly and said, "Come and have a cup of tea with me and I'll tell you what Reiki is."

So I sat down with him in the store. I was unsure and nervous because I didn't know what to expect. But the man's friendly manner put me at ease.

He explained to me: "Reiki was invented and developed by Dr. Usui in Japan. By allowing the energy of the universe to flow through your hands, you can heal yourself and other people or animals by laying hands on them. In doing so, you make use of the energy that is present in everything. The first step is to have the energy channels of your own body cleansed and corrected by a Reiki master. This is known as initiation. Together with the explanations, this is the first Reiki degree that you can acquire. With this you can help and heal yourself. Then there are higher Reiki levels, in which you also learn, for example, to give long-distance Reiki and to heal people who are in another city or even in another country. There are even special hospitals where only doctors and medical assistants who practise Reiki work," the Reiki master explained.

The friendly man took a lot of time for me and also told me that his life had changed for the better in all areas since he started practicing Reiki. I found him likeable, and with his eloquent way of speaking he quickly convinced me to take the first Reiki level with him. For the initiation, I was asked to sit upright on a chair, close my eyes and concentrate on my breathing. The master moved his hands along my body at some distance and explained to me in between that he was now correctly aligning the energy pathways along my spine. After about ten minutes, the procedure ended and he then showed me where I could apply Reiki myself in the future. At the end, I paid 250 rupees and received a booklet with teaching materials.

I had spent a whole two hours with the Reiki master and left him with the hope that I now had a new remedy in the fight against my headaches. I seriously wanted to try it out, practise Reiki every day from now on and heal myself. It was definitely worth a try - what did I have to lose? However, even after a few weeks of daily use, this attempt brought no improvement.

Over the next few days, I felt ill and weak. The weather was damp, sometimes rainy and quite chilly. I spent a lot of time in my dreary hotel room, which was only furnished with a bed with a rusty bed frame, a rickety white plastic table and matching chairs. No one had washed the curtains for years.

Occasionally I spoke to some of the people in my guesthouse. Among them was an Austrian my age. He told me that he had visited Shimla before and that you could buy and smoke hash everywhere there as it was grown in the mountainous region. He seemed to be quite a hardcore stoner. He even kept a dream diary that he used every morning after waking up so that he could tell the difference between dreams and reality. With some pride, I told him that I had been to Kashmir and smoked black Kashmiri hash. If I wasn't mistaken, he then saw me a little more respectful. We spent an evening together with some English people in their room. We told each other travel stories and the others smoked a joint. I abstained that evening. I knew that I was already limited in terms of conversation due to my pain. I didn't want to close myself off from the conversation even more by smoking a joint.

A British woman did most of the talking and I found her exciting and attractive. I had never met such a cool English woman before. She had traveled a lot and had had great adventures. However, I found it difficult to follow her lively explanations with a British accent. Although my English had improved enormously since my arrival, I couldn't tell any long stories because of my headaches and neck pain. They blocked my thinking and speaking too much. I would have liked to get to know the young woman better, but I simply didn't have the skills or the linguistic means to initiate this in any way. Such situations frustrated me. They made me feel inferior because I couldn't keep up with the others rhetorically. Worst of all, I could no longer impress girls I found interesting.

Otherwise, I spent the days alone and slept a lot. I went for daily walks through the town, but I was always exhausted quickly. I also bought pills for the stomach cramps and something for dehydration from a pharmacy.

Of course, I also visited the Dalai Lama's residence and was disappointed to find that he was traveling. What a shame, because I would have loved to meet this special person and see him up close. I had read in the Lonely Planet that you could take meditation courses at a Tibetan meditation center in Dharamsala. As I was very interested in this, I walked up the mountain to the center, which was a bit out of the way. After a while I found it and met a western-looking nun at the entrance. I had never spoken to a Buddhist nun before and felt unsure how to approach her.

"Hello," I finally said, "I would like to do a meditation course. Is that possible?".

"Hello," the nun replied, somewhat surprised, and explained to me: "A meditation course is currently running. It's been running for a few days and unfortunately it's not possible to join in the middle of it."

"Oh, that's a shame," I replied, somewhat disappointed. "And when does the next course start?".

"In three weeks."

"Hm, that's probably too late for me." After a pause, I asked: "Do you live here in the meditation center?"

"I'm from Australia and I'm here for six months every year. I spend the other half of the year in Australia, she replied with a warm smile."

"Oh, wow, interesting!".

As I didn't know what else to say or ask, I thanked her and left the meditation center, heading back downhill towards the town center. On the way back, I briefly considered whether I wanted to wait three weeks until the next course started. I really wanted to do a meditation course. On the other hand, I wanted to see more of India and spend the next few weeks traveling.

Indian hospitality

On the houseboat, I had met a group of travelers who had undertaken a pilgrimage to a particular mountain. Harjesh, a young man my age, had invited me to visit his family. They lived north of Delhi near Chandigarh. I accepted this opportunity and traveled on from Dharamsala. He lived with two siblings and his parents in a two-room apartment. They belonged there probably to the middle class. Although his parents didn't speak English, they were extremely hospitable. Over the next few days, I was introduced to the whole family, consisting of countless uncles, aunts and cousins. Everyone welcomed me warmly, and each time I was served cookies and Coca-Cola or a proper meal of rice, dal and chapatis.

I was deeply impressed by the high value placed on

family in India and the respect the children showed towards their parents. The longer I observed them, the more I realized that I unfortunately didn't have a good relationship with my parents, that we only spoke to each other a little and often argued.

A lasting impression

During the seven weeks in India, the pain was unfortunately a constant companion after the initial two days of pain relief. In addition, my stomach problems worsened due to a bacterial infection. As a result, I lost ten kilograms of weight during the seven weeks. At a height of 1.85 meters, I shrank from 70 kilograms to 60 kilograms. It looked a bit scary. My cheekbones now stood out exaggeratedly in front of my sunken cheeks. Even my knee joint now looked disproportionate in contrast to my thin legs.

Nevertheless, India made a deep and lasting impression on me. After an acclimatization phase, I had overcome my culture shock and started to notice aspects other than poverty and garbage. In addition, the solitude and isolation from everyday life in Germany made me reflect extensively on my previous life. I realized that in
India, family cohesion was one of the highest values in life and how much children valued and respected their parents, even though they had much less freedom than a teenager in Germany. They were not allowed to go to discos or drink alcohol, and there didn't seem to be any wild parties either. Relationships between men and women were only socially permitted if you got married. As long as you weren't married, you lived under the same roof as your parents. I decided to follow the example of valuing parents and family and to value my parents and my family more when I came back. I became more and more aware of how badly I had

behaved in the past. And deep down, I actually knew that my parents only ever wanted the best for me.

The strong faith of the Indians also left a lasting impression on me. Most of them were very devout, and you could see that everywhere. It was reflected in unmissable things like the countless temples or the many holy sadhus. But it was also evident in the little things of everyday life. Almost every tuk-tuk and every cab had a small figurine or picture of the gods Ganesh, Vishnu or Shiva in the driver's cabin. The figures were decorated with fresh, colorful flowers every day. The Indians also firmly believed in rebirth and karma. What sounded exotic to me was a matter of course for them: they believed that all the deeds you committed not only had an influence on this life, but also on subsequent lives in other incarnations. I realized that if you really believed this, as practically all Indians do, then it probably changed your perspective and attitude to life considerably. This is unavoidable because you have to plan for the long term - not just for one life, but for many lives. At least that's how the people I spoke to seemed to think. In terms of my pain, the trip to India hadn't been a breakthrough. But still I had the feeling that I had taken something valuable with me from this country, even if I couldn't quite grasp it yet.

STUDYING IN KIEL - THE DOWNHILL SLIDE CONTINUES

Start of studies

While I was still on my trip to India, I received some good news from my mother. She had the task of opening my mail while I was away. She told me that I had been offered a place to study business administration at Kiel University of Applied Sciences. I was lucky, because this course actually had a numerus clausus of 1.8, and my Abi average was 2.5. However, some of the places were allocated by lottery, and I had been lucky.

Just two days after my return, I went to Kiel to enrol in person. Two weeks later, I started a preparatory math course. I wanted to move into a shared flat with Kiki to study. Kiki was a good friend from our clique. But as we couldn't move into the apartment until October, I drove to Kiel every day for a week. The journey took an hour and a half. I had to leave at 7.00 a.m. so that I would be there in time for 9.00 a.m.. In the morning, I was always fighting against a leaden tiredness, so that I sometimes had little second lapses while driving. Fortunately, everything went well.

I was looking forward to sharing a flat with Kiki. My own apartment for the first time! Finally, the stress with my parents would stop and I would be my own boss. I had been good friends with Kiki for about three years. She was one grade level below me and we often hung out together. We often philosophized for hours at parties. She was going to start studying literature at university.

However, I was worried about my state of health. It hadn't got any better since my stay in India. The headaches and neck pain accompanied me throughout the day. I had problems expressing myself and my mood fluctuated between irritable and frustrated. I imagined what it would be like in this state in Kiel. Would I even be able to follow the subject matter? And more importantly, would I be able to make new friends at the university?

I had the feeling that a certain distance had already developed between me and some of my old friends. It seemed to me that I was no longer particularly pleasant company. That's why I couldn't hold it against anyone personally; it was just the way things were and I blamed the tension in my neck. I hated that tension to the core. I hated the pressure in my temples. I was angry that I was behaving the way I was behaving. Everything that went wrong in my life had its origins in this tension in my neck. The neck was the epicenter of all evil and negativity. And it seemed to keep going downhill.

Basically, I found it easier to be with old friends. I had a kind of "Past bonus". If I had a bad day, it was tolerated as a phase. But finding new friends in that state would be extremely difficult. Before getting involved in a new friendship, the "candidate" was always scrutinized for a while. I wouldn't have given myself a good report card. My self-confidence had suffered an enormous slump. I was no longer the same carefree Philip that I was two years ago. I did feel that I still had positive potential somewhere inside me. Unfortunately, it was just buried deep down because of this shitty pain.

I was able to put my reservations to the test in the preliminary course. The material wasn't easy, but it wasn't very complicated. I had already covered all of this at school, even if I had forgotten some of it. Basic math had been my best subject at school. I didn't find math really exciting, but the teacher had managed to get it across well and I didn't find it too difficult. In the preliminary course, I quickly realized that I could still follow the lecturer to some extent despite the headache. During the breaks, I even managed to have an almost normal conversation with some of the people sitting next to me a few times. But there were also other breaks when I didn't know what to do with myself, didn't want to stand anywhere and felt a bit uncomfortable. As the week drew to a close, I found that my worst fears were not confirmed, but neither were they invalidated. It remained to be seen how everything would develop.

Acupuncture

As my head and neck pain continued to be a constant companion, I decided to try a new doctor a few weeks after moving to Kiel. This time I chose an orthopaedist who also offered acupuncture. During my community service, an old lady had told me that the acupuncture sessions had significantly alleviated her knee pain. I was hoping for a similar effect. As I had already exhausted the so-called conservative therapy measures at the previous orthopaedist without success, the doctor admitted me for the acupuncture sessions. The health insurance company paid for eight sessions as part of a study. Two or three times I actually felt a little better for a few hours after a session, but that was it.

When the last of the eight acupuncture sessions came and the doctor wanted to insert the needles, I turned to him: "Doctor, this is my last session, and so far, unfortunately, there has only sometimes been a short-term improvement directly after the treatment. After one night, however, the positive effect is completely gone again every time."

The doctor replied: "Hm, you have exhausted all conservative treatment options. If acupuncture hasn't helped either, I don't know what to do. Then you'll probably have to live with the pain."

I thought I didn't hear correctly! I was about to reply:

"If that's the case, I'll probably take my own life sooner or later, because I can't stand it much longer!" But at the last moment, I decided not to answer. Who knows: maybe they would put me in a closed institution otherwise. But I was so angry!

'How can a doctor say something like that to his patient? That was an indictment! They should revoke his license,' my thoughts flashed through my head.

I had already consulted four doctors about my head and neck problems.

The first was my family doctor, who adjusted my neck several times. Afterwards, I read in my internet research that this was a controversial treatment.

Secondly, the first orthopaedist prescribed me physiotherapy, which was so painful that I stopped the treatment.

The third was the orthopaedist who, after various unsuccessful therapeutic measures, advised me to drink a beer more often to relieve the tension.

The fourth was this doctor who told me that I would have to live with this pain for the rest of my life.

At this point, my trust in doctors was shaken to the core

for the first time. I decided to inform myself even more intensively and find the right therapies myself. Apparently, you couldn't rely on the doctors!

Many hours of internet research later I had found out that I had actually tried the classic therapeutic approaches. The next step would have been pain therapy with antidepressants to counteract the process of pain chronification. However, I realized at the same time that it was perhaps already far too late for this measure. I had had a headache every day for over a year and a half - even every minute I was awake. If I had received this tip or a referral to a pain therapist from my second orthopaedic surgeon eight months ago, I might have been spared a lot. I couldn't understand how a well-trained doctor could act so negligently. His behavior may have been partly responsible for the deterioration in my quality of life. The same goes for the orthopaedic surgeon in Kiel. Instead of telling me that I would have to live with the pain, he should have referred me to a pain therapist immediately to counteract the chronification of the pain. Once the pain had become chronic, it was difficult to reverse the process. You could also read about this on the internet - but no doctor had ever thought it necessary to tell me.

So it was high time I looked for a pain therapist.

Student life

The first few weeks at the university of applied sciences were a phase of reorientation for me. Most of the lessons in the first semester took place in class. This made it a little easier to get to know other people, as there were only about 40 people in a class.

But that doesn't mean it was easy for me. I had days when my head and neck hurt so much that I didn't feel able to hold a conversation. Such Days were bad, and they became more and more frequent. Nevertheless, to my surprise, I managed to make friends with Konrad and Suse. They had come to Kiel as a couple from Swabia because you could get a so-called double degree in Kiel. If you attended courses at a partner university abroad for a year, you would receive a Spanish and a German diploma, for example.

In our eight-storey UAS building, the business students occupied the bottom four floors, while the top four were taken up by the social studies students. You could usually tell at first glance which group someone belonged to. The business students wore checked shirts tucked into their trousers with sailor shoes, and the social work students tended to dress in wide corduroy pants and baggy looks with piercings. When I spent the break in the courtyard with Konrad and Suse, we looked much more like the social studies students. I had been wearing dreadlocks again for a while, and Konrad also stood out from the crowd of business students with his plait. Suse was recognizable by her wild brown mane of curls. Konrad and Suse both looked rather alternative. I really liked that.

I had a good chat with Konrad about music. He was into electronic music, especially Detroit techno and Schranz. That didn't suit my taste one hundred percent, but at least it was electronic music and I could relate to it. We started exploring the Kiel electro scene together. The two of them soon became my best friends at university and I really liked them. Apart from that, I knew a few people who I talked to from time to time, but overall I didn't have many connections there. The breaks were actually the worst thing for me because I felt isolated and like a failure because I hardly had any friends. If I hadn't at least had Konrad and Suse, I might even have dropped out of university.

Pain therapy

Two weeks after my last acupuncture session, I had an appointment with a doctor in Kiel who specializes in neurology, psychiatry and pain therapy. I felt extremely uncomfortable as I walked across the large square towards the practice. If I met an acquaintance and he asked me what I was doing here, what would I say? That I was on my way to a pain therapist, a psychiatrist? Certainly not! I thought about who lived in this neighborhood. There were quite a few, and the practice wasn't far from the center. You could always meet someone here. Maybe I could say I had a dentist appointment somewhere around here. But if I was then asked for his name and address, I would have a problem. Hopefully I would be spared that. And so a silly carousel of worries about my reputation spun in my head.

When I finally stood in front of the practice and read the sign, I felt quite queasy: "Doctor for neurology, psychiatry and pain therapy", it said. I'd been feeling strange all morning anyway, as if I had a slightly elevated temperature and was coming down with a cold. I was exhilarated and a bit woozy; the headache was also much less than usual today. The door was locked. I rang the bell to be let in. After climbing the stairs to the second floor, I was completely out of breath. My heart was pounding in my throat because now I had that fear again. Hopefully I would be able to get a meaningful word out to the doctor's receptionist. But they probably know a lot worse patients here than me, I thought. Real crazy people. But maybe I was one of them by now? To get into the practice, I had to ring the bell again. 'My God,' I thought, 'do they have to protect themselves from psychopaths like this, or why all the security measures?'

In the waiting room, the anxiety and fear continued. I had never particularly liked visits to the doctor, but since I had developed this illness, I hated them. Because I had to reveal something about myself, even though I had built up a thick protective shell around myself. I didn't want anyone to know how bad I really was, otherwise everyone would give me a wide berth. I filled in the medical history form that the receptionist had given me. For alcohol consumption I entered "occasionally", for drug consumption I wrote "marijuana occasionally between the ages of 16 and 19, no longer today". Both of these were somewhat embellished, but at least I didn't leave anything out. I only drank alcohol at the weekend and smoking weed had become increasingly rare. I usually only did it on special occasions, and when I did, I only took a few puffs on a joint. Since I used to smoke bong heads every other day, you could say that my consumption was hardly worth mentioning in comparison.

I estimated the doctor to be in her late 40s and, to my relief, I found her likeable. I tried to explain the history of my illness to her. I started with the snowboarding accident and explained what treatment I had undergone so far. To my astonishment, I had no major problems talking. I didn't have a shaky voice, nor did I have to struggle for words, and I was able to explain everything to her reasonably well. That's why I was immediately worried that she wouldn't even notice how bad I really was if I behaved so well.

I therefore emphasized that the headaches had already been pretty bad for me and were severely affecting my whole life. I also mentioned that I had problems concentrating at university. However, I kept quiet about my intense stoner past and the panic attacks. It was just too embarrassing and too personal for me, and I didn't feel much like talking about it.

Fortunately, she didn't ask any more questions. That was very good for me.

Meanwhile, the doctor made notes on her computer. Then a doctor's assistant carried out some tests on me. She measured my brain waves with a device that looked a bit like a mind-reading cap from a science fiction movie. She also took my blood. I was then called back into the doctor's treatment room.

She described my symptoms in roughly the same way as I had read on the internet: "Your brain waves are fine, the blood test is still being carried out, but overall it can be said that you have already experienced pain chronification. Do you know what pain chronification is or how it comes about?"

"Uh, probably, I've read quite a bit about it, but feel free to explain it again."

She then started talking for quite a while about neurotransmitters, endorphins, habituation effects and a vicious circle that got worse and worse until finally they were talking about a pain disorder. There was a lot I didn't understand, but by large her presentation was in line with what I had already read.

"As a therapy, I will prescribe you tricyclic antidepressants in low doses. They counteract pain chronification and also have a calming, sedative and slightly mood-enhancing effect."

She took a packet of tablets out of her cupboard and gave them to me. "The active ingredient is called amitriptyline. It's the usual remedy for chronic pain to counteract the vicious circle of pain and tension. And it would also be very useful to learn a relaxation technique to combat muscle tension."

She recommended a book on progressive muscle relaxation according to Jacobsen and gave me an exercise cassette to go with it.

I was told to start with 20 milligrams of amitriptyline. The doctor explained to me that side effects such as dry mouth, nervousness and tiredness could occur, especially at the beginning of the treatment.

"How long do you think I'll have to take this medication?" I asked.

"In many cases, drug treatment can be discontinued after around six months," she replied.

That sounded good to me. I really wanted to take the stuff that was supposed to manipulate my brain for as short a time as possible. I didn't have a particularly positive attitude towards antidepressants. It felt a bit like failure to me to have to take them. You couldn't manage in this life without chemical substances of your own accord. That seemed like a flaw to me, and you couldn't tell anyone because many people would label you as a psycho.

Above all, however, I was extremely happy to have finally found someone who seemed to understand my symptoms and also knew what to do about them. After the visit to the doctor, new hope sprouted in me and taking Amitriptyline brought about a phenomenal change! The headaches were almost gone after just three days! I could articulate myself again to some extent and the right words came to me again at the right time. I became downright euphoric. I hoped that all the suffering would now come to a quick end and I would be back to my old self.

However, I also felt the side effects that the doctor had mentioned. My mouth was often as dry as the Sahara desert. In some situations, it could get so bad that I could no longer speak - especially in situations where I got nervous. And unfortunately there were plenty of those. So from then on, I made sure that I always had enough sweets in my mouth to avoid unnecessary embarrassment. The tiredness was already plaguing me increased by a few degrees. I found it even harder to get out of bed in the morning and was still so tired at the lectures that I often almost fell off my chair. It wasn't unusual for me to sleep for twelve hours straight at the weekend. I also had the impression that the tablets made me even more listless, although the absence of pain naturally opened up a lot of new possibilities for me.

Unfortunately, the wonderful effect of being pain-free only lasted for two weeks. After that, the headaches came back slowly but steadily and got a little worse every day. When I returned to the practice six weeks later, the effect had faded more and more. The doctor therefore decided to increase the dosage. After this increase, the pain subsided again for a while. But then a kind of tolerance seemed to gradually build up again and the pain level increased again. I became disillusioned. Amitriptyline was therefore not the miracle cure it had initially seemed to be.

Progressive muscle relaxation

Following the doctor's recommendation, I bought the book on muscle relaxation according to Jacobsen by Wilhelm Johnen. In the introduction to my 1995 edition from the GU publishing house it said: "Jacobsen recognized that through targeted tensing and abrupt release of individual muscle groups, improved relaxation - both physical and psychological - can be demonstrably achieved. With regular training, you gain the ability to positively influence your mental balance: you become more balanced, can meet the demands of an increasingly demanding working world more calmly and your self-confidence grows."

It sounded good and I was able to confirm the effects. Progressive muscle relaxation alleviated my suffering at least a little. I took half an hour almost every day, closed my bedroom door and did the relaxation exercise with the exercise cassette. I tensed one muscle area at a time, then relaxed it again, felt into it for a while and went through the whole body. As a result, my muscles gradually relaxed more and more deeply. I felt noticeably better after such a session, even if the effect usually only lasted for two to three hours. So on some days I did two sessions.

Now, for the first time, I had an instrument to improve my own condition and actively fight the pain. As a weapon in the fight against pain, however, it had little firepower. It was more like a pistol than a machine gun. I managed to inflict moderate losses on the enemy army of pain and even pushed it back a little for a short time. But that was nowhere near enough to permanently weaken the troops, win a battle, let alone win an entire war for me. Nevertheless, it was much more than a drop in the ocean and made my everyday life a little easier.

Your own four walls

The first few weeks in my own apartment were cool, but only if you ignore the pain. Because I didn't really enjoy anything anymore. Nevertheless, it was an interesting experience to be the master of my own home. I could cook my favorite meal every day and sleep as late as I wanted at the weekend without anyone complaining. I could smoke weed whenever I felt like it and didn't have to worry about being caught in this broad state or meeting annoying parents. However, I no longer smoked pot as often, mainly at the weekend in combination with alcohol on special occasions. In the meantime, I had the feeling that the neck tension and headaches under the influence of marijuana were even more intense and unpleasant than usual. I now often felt very unwell when I was flat, especially when I had smoked weed in company. Sometimes I couldn't formulate a single sensible sentence afterwards. I also suspected that smoking weed was at least a contributing factor to my illness.

Attempts to cope with everyday life

I had already pressed 'snooze' three times on the alarm clock. If I wanted to get to my first lecture on time, I had to hurry now. Dazed, I sat down on the edge of the bed. Getting up was the first pain of the day. My neck felt stiff and uncomfortable and my head was pounding. I had also had a bad dream. I trotted towards the bathroom, then into the kitchen, quickly made myself a strong coffee and a chocolate muesli with milk, devoured it hastily and then jogged to the bus stop. After a short wait, the bus to the college arrived. It was quite full and, as usual, I only got a standing room only seat at first. Only after a few stops did the seats empty out and there were mainly students left. The university was on the outskirts of the city on the eastern bank of the fjord.

I had a long day today, two hours of economics, two hours of statistics, then two hours of law, and two hours of English in the late afternoon. When I got off the bus, the queasy feeling in my stomach intensified. I wanted to get back on the bus and drive on. My body and my subconscious rebelled. They wanted to not to enter the university area. The idea alone made me feel uncomfortable. I had to force myself.

I sat down in an empty seat in the lecture hall and was glad that no one approached me so early in the morning. During the lecture, I fought against tiredness. A few times my eyes closed briefly. There were times when I couldn't follow the material. That was always the case in the morning. The tiredness only subsided around midday.

During the first break, I went to the IT room on the second floor to surf the internet. I didn't feel able to have meaningful conversations with my fellow students today and wanted to avoid it. At lunchtime, I went to the canteen on my own. I didn't have a fixed lunch group. Konrad and

Suse rarely ate in the canteen, they cooked a lot at home and didn't live far from the university campus.

On the way to the canteen, I met some fellow students, but tried to avoid them so as not to have to talk to them - too exhausting. I wonder what they thought I was eating alone again. They probably thought I was a freak who didn't have any friends. That wasn't so far from the truth. I still found it difficult to socialize.

As I stood waiting in the food queue, Marco happened to stand behind me. He was in my semester and we had already spoken briefly a few times.

"Hello, how are you?" said Marco.

"Thank you, I am good. What are you doing here?" I replied. I always had the feeling that I was lying to people when I answered the question about how I was feeling. I wasn't feeling well at all, on the contrary, I was feeling really bad. But it was just a phrase. Nobody in the canteen queue wanted to know about my pain odyssey and certainly not about the fact that it was hurting right now. It was just too negative. I wonder if he had heard from my tone of voice that I wasn't feeling as well as I had claimed. And why did I actually asked what he was doing here? It was obvious that he wanted lunch.

"I was just in the law lecture and now I'm really hungry."

"Uh, yeah, me too."

There was a somewhat awkward pause in the conversation. I couldn't think of anything else to say and looked down at the floor. I could clearly feel the unpleasant pressure on my temples.

"Is there anything tasty today? I forgot to look at the menu overview at the entrance," Marco then asked.

I had looked at the menu at the entrance. Of the three menus, I only liked the one I had chosen. But I couldn't remember the names of the two menus I didn't like nor the menu I had actually chosen. The pain overrode everything and my brain didn't want to spit anything out. The information just wasn't accessible. "Uh, I don't know, I didn't look at it either," I lied.

"What did you do at the weekend? Was there a good party somewhere?" Marco asked after another tough pause in the conversation.

"No party this time. I was at the studio movie theater."

"What movie have you seen?"

I thought about what the movie was called, but I couldn't think of it. I remembered that I quite liked it, but I only had a vague idea of the plot.

"Hm ... I can't think of the title right now."

"Which actors were involved?"

I certainly couldn't remember the names of the actors.

"I don't know," I replied.

Another pause in the conversation. I was embarrassed that once again I had no idea about anything!

"It was about some crazy guy, American movie. It was quite good."

A meaningless answer, but at least I had managed to get some kind of reaction.

Situations like this happened all the time: that I actually knew something, but couldn't access the information in conversational situations because I was so tense. And that constantly gnawed away at my self-confidence. I couldn't have a sensible conversation. And while others in a group were talking about their opinions and drawing attention to themselves, I usually hid quietly in the background so as not to expose myself.

The queue continued and I grabbed a tray and dishes. I hesitated briefly: should I ask Marco if we wanted to eat together? Or do I wait for him after the food is served?

At the same moment, I saw Florian and Henning sitting in the canteen, with whom Marco usually hung out. Then he'll certainly join them, I thought. After getting myself some tortellini with cream sauce, I quickly moved on and made my way to the other corner of the canteen so that I didn't pass Florian and Henning. I knew them too well not to say hello and too badly not to join them at the lunch table.

I sat down alone at a table and started to eat. After a while, I saw that Marco had actually sat down with Florian and Henning and all three of them were chatting animatedly. I was envious of the group and at the same time glad that I was sitting alone in peace and didn't have to talk to anyone. After lunch, I went back to the main building on my own and had two more hours of English. I was already exhausted. A normal day, but it felt like running the gauntlet.

When I got home that afternoon, I threw myself on my bed and slept for an hour from exhaustion.

After a while, the daily routine of studying almost overwhelmed me.

Getting out of bed in the morning was like an ordeal. I felt woozy and drowsy after every night. Although I drank strong coffee for breakfast, this state lasted most of the morning. The morning lectures were usually one big battle against sleep for me. It took an enormous amount of energy for me to even keep my eyes open, let alone follow the subject matter sufficiently. This kind of tiredness was definitely not normal. As a result, I often slept through the first lecture and only made it to the second.

The enormous tiredness seemed to be related to the tablets I had been prescribed, but also somehow to my condition. With the constant headaches, everything took a lot more energy. Of the 100 percent of my attention that was normally available, 70 percent was occupied with the pain. I had the remaining 30 percent available to, for example, drive a car and correctly assess the traffic, follow complicated study content or simply have a conversation with a fellow student. In order to achieve a reasonably satisfactory result in such activities, I had to be many times more concentrated and motivated, simply because I only had 30 percent of my mental resources at my disposal.

This "operating mode" took a lot of energy. Sleeping increasingly became my favorite activity. I found sleep relieving because I didn't feel the pain while I slept. I didn't have to endure any suffering and the negative thoughts fell silent. Every day I longed for evening to come and I could finally leave this day full of pain and suffering behind me. In bed, I could slip into a state where I could escape this hell for a while. The same applied to the weekend, when I got so drunk at parties that the pain became bearable and faded into the background. It didn't disappear then completely, but the alcohol at least partially suppressed it. When I saw homeless people getting drunk on the street, I could suddenly understand why they were doing it: because they couldn't bear their own suffering and wanted to numb themselves. Alcohol was their "medicine for forgetting". I could understand how you could slowly slip into such a situation without really being able to do anything about it. I hoped I would be spared this fate.

Increasing the dose

I visited the pain therapist regularly every two to three months and reported on my condition. The doctor kept increasing the dosage until we had reached 100 milligrams. After each increase, I felt a little better for a while until the effect wore off. With this high dosage, however, my symptoms stabilized at a low level. I could now tolerate the headaches a little better than a few months ago, but they still restricted me in every everyday situation. It just didn't seem to be going any further downhill with the medication. They stopped the downhill slide. However, I was already in a deep, deep hellhole and wanted to get out of it. However, it didn't look as if the tablets could reverse the pain chronification and free me from the pain. Sometimes I thought that maybe opiates would be the right painkillers for me. I had read that they were supposed to be stronger. However, they also had the disadvantage of being addictive.

It was foreseeable that the pain would accompany me for the next few years and that I would not be able to get off this medication so quickly. In addition to the other side effects, the higher dosage also caused constipation. Although I had calculated that this therapy would give me a really good chance, my new hope of a better life without pain died once again. And this was already therapy attempt number five. It was maddening!

Biofeedback

After it became clear that increasing the dosage of tablets was not having any significant effect, I asked if there were any other treatment options. The doctor then told me about biofeedback and behavioral therapy.

She referred me to a psychologist she knew. After a long conversation, he said that behavioral therapy would probably not be too helpful for my symptoms. I would still be able to cope relatively well in everyday life. Apparently, I had once again given too positive an impression during our conversation. But he gave me an introduction to biofeedback and gave me a portable biofeedback device to take home with me so that I could use it every day. I stuck the electrodes to my temples and neck and the device produced sounds. When I tensed and relaxed the muscles, the sounds changed, so you could train yourself to relax.

However, even after practicing daily for weeks, I had hardly any success. Progressive muscle relaxation continued to have a greater effect than biofeedback. I therefore also stopped this therapy without any results - that was attempt number six.

Botox

The psychologist then suggested that I take part in a study. At the pain clinic in Kiel, they were currently testing botulinum toxin as a medication for migraines and Tension headaches. It is also known as Botox. Rich and famous people in particular like to have it injected to smooth out their facial wrinkles. I called the number the psychologist had given me and got an appointment in three weeks. The clinic was right next to the college. I filled out a lot of questionnaires and was then injected with Botox in my temples and neck. It was supposed to paralyze the muscles a little, relax them and thus reduce the pain. So much for the theory. I was to receive two injections 3 months apart. As this was a double-blind study, neither I nor my doctor knew whether I was receiving the real medication or a placebo for the first injection. For the second injection, I would definitely get the Botox. A few weeks after the first injection, it seemed to me that there had been some improvement. On the study questionnaire, I reported a "20 percent improvement". A few months later, however, I put it down to the placebo effect. Once again, I had placed a lot of hope and expectations in this treatment method. That's probably why the placebo effect was relatively strong.

Even after the second injection, my condition had hardly changed. According to the doctor treating me, the result of the study was that there was a slight improvement in migraines, but no significant improvement in tension headaches. At the end of the two treatment sessions, I still had the familiar headaches. This was trial number seven.

New Year's Eve in Kiel

We celebrated New Year's Eve with Kiki and me in our shared flat in Kiel-Gaarden. From my room I had a great view of Kiel's west bank and was able to enjoy the fireworks over the city. Friends and acquaintances from Kiel, from our old home in Dithmarschen, from Flensburg and Lübeck came together, and we had a party of about 15 people. We had a pre-party throughout the evening, and there was a lot of smoking, bong smoking and large quantities of alcohol consumed. Pretty drunk, we made our way to the Max with a few other people. It was a large disco in Kiel where you could party quite well. It was an exuberant evening and as I was so drunk that I hardly felt my pain and anxiety any more, I felt quite exhilarated and free surrounded by friends.

At some point when it was already late at night, I had lost everyone and seemed to be the only one of our clique still in the Max. I decided to make my way home as well. As I was leaving the disco, I noticed a particularly pretty dark-haired girl who was also just leaving. In my normal state, I would never have dared to do that - and if I had, I wouldn't have been able to think of anything to say. But in my drunken, exhilarated state, I approached her:

"Hello, I wish you a happy new year! Did you have a good party? Can I keep you company for a little while on the way?"

"Yes, I had a good party, but that's enough now. It's getting late and I'm going home," the girl replied with an Eastern European accent.

I continued: "I was celebrating with my friends, but now

I couldn't find them. They've probably already gone home. But they're actually all sleeping in my shared flat. Well, now I'll have to see how I can get home on my own. Tell me, you have such a nice-sounding accent. Where are you from? Are you here in Kiel to study?"

"I come from Poland and work here as an au pair."

"Ah, then you can probably drink more vodka than me!" I tried to tease her and laughed. "That's why you still look so sober, because you're so hardened. You've probably drunk a lot more than I have! And I drank quite a lot. I didn't count every glass, but it wasn't a small amount. In any case, we had a great evening!"

Now she had to laugh: "I very rarely drink vodka. I only had a couple of beers today and a sparkling wine to toast at midnight."

"And how is life as an au pair? Did you get any nice kids or do they annoy you all day?"

"Oh, they're great! I look after a four-year-old girl and a three-year-old boy. We play a lot and have a good relationship."

"I could do with an au pair to play with me from time to time. I think you'd be just the right person," I grinned at her.

"I think you've already passed the age limit for that," she replied with amusement."

"Oh, that's a shame," I replied with slightly feigned disappointment. Tell me, where are we actually going, I don't know my way around here. Do you remember where we are?"

"My au pair family's house is just around the corner. We are close to Schrevenpark."

I dropped her off at the front door and got her name and phone number. Her name was Anuschka. Elated and proud, I made my way home. As I was still a long way from our apartment and kept getting lost, I finally hailed a cab and got a ride home.

The next day I lounged around on the couch all day because I felt sick to my stomach from all the alcohol. But I felt happier and more alive today than I had in the last few months. The headaches were always much less the next day after a night of drinking. I put this down to the mood-lifting effect of the alcohol, which boosted endorphin production.

The day after next my stomach felt healthy again. I overcame my fears and called Anuschka and we arranged to meet for a beer in the Irish pub. I didn't really have high hopes that she would still find me interesting when I was sober. I was already finding it difficult to keep a flowing conversation going or maintain eye contact. I only forced a laugh when I thought it was appropriate. I certainly wasn't a very entertaining conversation partner for a girl in my condition, I thought. But I had to try anyway, I owed it to myself as a man, after all I hadn't even had sex for almost two years.

I was quite nervous when I was waiting for her in the pub. I also had problems with my dry mouth because of the antidepressants. But I'd always had sweets with me recently. When Anushka finally arrived, I was amazed to see that she was even prettier and more enchanting than I remembered. I went to great lengths to present myself in a good light. At least I managed to avoid major pauses in conversation. Moreover, I only stuttered occasionally and somewhat gallantly disguised my word-finding difficulties. All in all, the evening turned out to be quite nice. However, I didn't manage to recreate the sizzling atmosphere from New Year's Eve. As I suspected, she had no further interest in getting to know me after that.

I was now able to record a new negative experience for myself and my frustration about my condition and my current living environment increased once again - just as small and larger new frustrations were added every day and made my life a little more difficult. Many things that were completely normal for other people were now out of reach for me.

Summer construction projects

Every year, my father carried out a summer building project to expand and modernize the farm. A new silo slab, a new stable building, a new milking parlor - he was always coming up with new ideas. During the summer semester break, I always spent a few weeks with my parents to help them with these building projects. I also used this opportunity to top up my Bafög.

My job was usually to mix the concrete mixes. My father had a large concrete mixer for this, which was hitched behind the tractor and driven by it. I filled the mixer with gravel, which I picked up from a pile of gravel with the shovel of the front loader tractor and then tipped into the mixer. By now I was quite adept at this and only poured a little gravel next to it. Then I climbed off the tractor and poured two bags of cement powder and several buckets of water into the mixer.

It was a physical job where you still had to be able to drive a bit of a tractor. It was a job that I could do reasonably well in my condition with the headaches. There wasn't much human interaction, I didn't have to perform in front of a group and I didn't have to be in a good mood. Perhaps it was my destiny to work on my father's farm after all. If I failed my studies or was unable to do another job due to my pain, that was still a possibility - an undesirable but not entirely unrealistic vision of the future. If that didn't work out either and I took the vision one step further, I found myself in a group home for mentally ill people. But I tried not to get too carried away with such thoughts.

I no longer argued with my father and mother as often as I did when I was still living with them. The distance, but also my visit to India and the insight, the fact that I hadn't exactly made their lives any easier with my behavior and complaints had improved the situation. I still found it difficult to have a meaningful conversation with my father. But at least the really big arguments were no longer the order of the day. The underlying tension in the air was also no longer so unbearable.

As far as my pain was concerned, I told my parents about my countless attempts at therapy and the failures and they showed understanding, compassion and gave tips and advice when they could think of something else to try. But basically they were quite helpless in the face of the whole issue. As far as my emotional situation was concerned, I shared much less with them. I didn't want to overwhelm them with the darkness that lay dormant inside me. They probably wouldn't have known what to do with it either.

Phenylalanine

As my trust in doctors had already been fundamentally shaken, I was constantly searching the internet for other alternative pain therapies. At one point, I came across the active ingredient phenylalanine. This is an amino acid and an endogenous precursor for endorphin production. Endorphin production is normally reduced in pain patients. The administration of phenylalanine can increase endorphin production, according to the product description. So I ordered 100 tablets from the Netherlands for 40 marks and tried my luck. I really didn't have much left to lose.

When I came back from a vacation with my friend Jens in Spain and Morocco, I started taking the tablets. Of course, I took them in addition to the amitriptyline. I soon noticed a strange effect.

My heart was beating much faster than usual, which didn't feel so healthy. However, there was also another decisive effect. The headache was gone! I was able to use a creative choice of words again and floated on a euphoric cloud for a whole week.

I had found a miracle cure! Why didn't any doctor know about it? I finally stopped taking my antidepressants in one fell swoop - and remained pain-free. Another week later, I had an appointment with my neurologist and told her about my success. She was skeptical and not at all thrilled that I had simply stopped taking the antidepressants. A week later, the headaches returned and I started taking the antidepressants again. The effect was gone. Once again.

It had been worth a try, but I acknowledged defeat. The disease just seemed invincible. My hope that I would ever be able to lead a halfway normal life again diminished a little. So I had arrived at attempt number eight.

Throughout my time of study and suffering in Kiel, I became increasingly interested in alternative medicine, as conventional medicine had so far only brought me failure and frustration. I bought as many books as I could on acupuncture, homeopathy, acupressure, spiritual healing and Reiki. I was also interested in esoteric books about the spiritual energy systems of the body, the chakras - as well as anything about mysticism, meditation, yoga and pain healing. My bookshelf was overflowing with such books and I spent a lot of time reading them. These topics fascinated me and I devoured the books. I was already thinking about whether I should pursue a career in this direction. After my studies, I thought, I could work in a business administration job for a few years and then train as a non-medical practitioner. Then I could focus on topics that were really close to my heart.

Support in the call center

In the second year of my studies, I worked part-time as a call center agent for a telecommunications provider. The call center was directly opposite our shared apartment, so I had an extremely short commute to work. My job was to help end customers who couldn't access the Internet or set up their email client themselves with the configuration.

I had sweated blood and water to get this job, because in the application and recruitment rounds you had to introduce yourself in front of the other applicants and the people from Freenet. Of course, this had triggered a few severe anxiety attacks in me again, but somehow I had finally fought my way through. Now I was actually doing a surprisingly good job, I thought. With friendliness and patience, I was able to compensate somewhat for my limited language skills on the phone. I also always had to ask a lot of questions and the explanations I had to give were often repetitive.

All in all, I was actually very fascinated by this IT world. The soft skills that were so highly praised everywhere and in which I almost invariably performed miserably were not so important here. What really mattered here was that you had the right knowledge to solve specific problems. I saw that I could also score points in this environment with my limited communication skills. I also liked the somewhat nerdy group of people. I therefore soon decided to focus my studies on information technologies.

During one of my Sunday shifts, I had already spent three hours and made a few phone calls when I decided to get a coffee from the kitchen.

"Hello," I said to the three boys who were standing in the kitchen chatting. No 'hello' came back. Maybe they were too engrossed in their conversation? Or maybe I wasn't important enough. Two of the boys were permanent employees who had a bit more to say - even if I didn't know exactly what position they actually held.

I took a coffee cup from the cupboard and put it in the coffee machine. While the coffee was being prepared, I wondered whether I should go and talk to the three of them. But what should I say, what should I talk to them about? I probably wouldn't get a word out or start saying something totally stupid.

Now the three of them started laughing out loud. Were they laughing at me? Had they perhaps made a joke about me that I hadn't noticed?

Although I had been working in this office for several months, I had never exchanged more than a few sentences with anyone there in all that time. At the start of my shift, I always found a seat of my choice, logged on to the telephone system and waited for a caller to come through. Some days we were on the phone almost non-stop; there was hardly any opportunity to talk to the person sitting next to us anyway. But there were also quiet days when you would have had plenty of time to talk to the person sitting next to you or walk around a bit and chat with others.

I'm sure the three boys thought I was a loner, a freak, a shy, weird, depressive person, someone with whom something was wrong. Someone you could take the piss out of and make fun of. Once again, I felt inferior. These thought patterns were extremely unpleasant. They paralyzed me and produced their own reality. But I couldn't turn them off at will either. Had I already become like this?

Was it a kind of paranoia?

When my coffee was ready, I quickly left the kitchen again - frustrated and frightened by the thoughts that were running around in my head.

Homeopathy

My mother had received a recommendation from an acquaintance for an alternative practitioner in Kiel who specialized in homeopathy and I wanted to give it a try. As the health insurance didn't cover the costs, I had to pay the fee myself. 180 marks for a two-hour anamnesis session and 50 marks per follow-up appointment. That was quite a lot of money, but as a poor student with a decent amount of student loans, I was lucky that my parents also supported me. They probably wanted to help me at least in this way because of my poor health, so that I didn't have financial worries on top of the pain. Besides, there is hardly a better investment than in your own health.

The naturopath practiced in her own home and I immediately felt at ease with her. She took a lot of time and asked me lots of questions about my habits, such as whether I preferred sweet or salty foods. She also wanted to know exactly what illnesses had occurred in my family, for example in my grandparents and their parents. She asked me to research this in more detail before my next appointment. It felt good that someone took so much time and tried to really understand my problem with so much understanding. For the first time I felt that my complaints were being taken seriously by a doctor. At the end of the appointment, she placed various homeopathic pellets, known as globules, on my hand one after the other. I was supposed to notice whether I felt any effect. However, I didn't feel anything and I was given a certain type of globules to take several times a day. I was also told to avoid alcohol, coffee and toothpaste containing iodine, as this would impair the effect. The toothpaste wasn't a problem, I considerably reduced my alcohol consumption for a few weeks, but I just couldn't give up coffee. Without coffee, I was simply not fit for everyday life.

Together with my mother, I researched our family tree to find out what illnesses had run in our family. They included Parkinson's, osteoporosis, diabetes and a few others. You could really get scared of old age. Somehow, every relative had had some terrible disease! At least our family DNA seemed to be cancer-free. With this information, I went back to the homeopath and she provided me with new, different globules. However, when these had no effect at all after a few more appointments and attempts, and I had already spent a lot of money on them, I was discouraged and stopped trying treatment number nine.

Hide and seek

The worst part of the whole time was that I had to hide my true self. I thought that the intensity of my negativity would overwhelm everyone. I couldn't imagine that anyone could come close to understanding it or have any lasting sympathy for my condition. At least I shared with my parents that this constant pain was tormenting me. But they only had a rudimentary idea of what my inner emotional life was really like. Most of the time, I played a role. I tried not to let all the suffering and negativity come out too much and not to let anyone really notice.

It turned out to be very strenuous to play this role, andI also found it sad that nobody actually knew the 'real' Philip. On the other hand, I couldn't imagine that anyone would want to be friends with the real Philip. I didn't like myself like that. I would have loved to run away from myself screaming! I was sure that if I had acted out my negative emotions, I would have driven my last friends away very quickly.

If I did try to tell someone about my condition, the first question I was usually asked was: "And did you go to the doctor?" This question alone almost sent me into a rage, as I thought it was so incredibly naive that I found it hard to bear. I had been trying to find a therapy that worked for years on the side, so to speak - so far without success. Most people assumed that doctors could cure everything except cancer and AIDS. Unfortunately, I didn't share this opinion at all. I had had other experiences.

I was met with so much incomprehension that I simply found it exhausting to deal with this knowledge gap with questions and answers. The few, discouraging attempts to share my true inner state with someone encouraged me to keep the whole story to myself. It was probably just too difficult for others to put themselves in my shoes as a healthy person. It also hurt tremendously every time I had to talk about my health, as the associated negative emotions were triggered and flooded my system.

BALI - IN THE PARADISE OF FRUSTRATION

Breakwater

On a windy day, I fought my way through the rough seas and kept an eye out for a suitable wave within reach. You had to catch it at the right moment to ride it. I'd been in the water for a while, but the smaller surfboard I'd swapped with my fellow student Lars for the afternoon was struggling and felt a bit wobbly. I hadn't really caught a wave yet today.

Suddenly I saw a gigantic wave rolling towards me. It reared up to a height of four meters in front of me and I felt extremely queasy at the sight. I already knew from my own experience over the last few months that big waves can really swirl you around and keep you underwater for a while if they break directly above you. I paddled my board towards the giant mountain, further out to sea. I wanted to climb the wave before it broke. I just managed to push myself over the crest of the wave at the last second and then fell into the depths.

An initial moment of relief quickly gave way to renewed

panic when I saw another wave of the same size and height rolling towards me. I wondered whether I should swim back towards it and try to climb it before it broke. When I looked back at the beach, however, I realized that I was already several hundred meters out in the open sea. With these huge waves and this current, it was dangerous, probably life-threatening.

So I turned around and tried to paddle towards the beach. But the current of the wave pulled back so strongly that I only just managed to paddle on the spot until the wave finally broke directly above me.

I was torn back and forth and thrown through the masses of water like a sock in a washing machine. I didn't know which way was up and which way was down and time stretched out like chewing gum. After a while, I started to run out of air and panic spread. I was still whirling back and forth. Since I didn't know which way was up and which way was down, I didn't know which way I could swim to surface.

I finally managed to push my head through the surface of the water and was able to take a breath. I felt relief and immediately looked around for my surfboard. I knew it couldn't be more than four meters away because of the leash on my leg. I spotted it three meters away from me, swam towards it, grabbed the board and took a quick breath. I was in shock because I felt that I had just escaped a life-threatening situation.

When I looked around, I could hardly believe my eyes. A third huge wave came rolling towards me, which looked just as high and powerful as the previous ones. I barely had time to paddle before it came at me again. I had the presence of mind to take another big breath, because I knew that I would be under water for another 30 to 40 seconds. Once again, I was grabbed by the enormous force of the wave and whirled around. It felt like torture to be underwater, not being able to breathe, not knowing where was up and where was down and not being able to estimate when the wave would release me again - or whether I would resurface in time before I ran out of air. I wondered what would happen if I had to breathe before I reached the surface. I imagined that the moment the breathing reflex kicked in and could no longer be stopped, the water would press into my lungs and I would die an agonizing death of drowning.

I finally made it to the surface and clung to my board again. This time, a normal-sized wave of around two and a half meters came at me rolled towards me. I realized that I was now very far out to sea and that it was probably my last chance to catch this wave and ride it towards the beach. I started to paddle. But I was shocked when I realized that my arms felt like rubber and had hardly any strength. I mobilized my very last reserves as I felt that my life was at stake here. Finally, I picked up enough speed to catch the wave. Lying on my stomach, I clung to the board and was swept towards the beach with the wave. The wave was so powerful that it carried me several hundred meters onto the beach. I was lucky that I kept my balance and didn't go into a spin.

I rolled off the board on the beach, haggard and unable to fully comprehend what had just happened. My whole body was shaking. There was a sign sticking out of the beach right in front of me with a skull and crossbones and the words "Strong currents, swimming prohibited".

In the meantime, my buddy had recognized my precarious situation and tried to get the lifeguards to help me. But they refused, saying that it would have been too dangerous for them in the swell. One of the fins on my buddy's board had broken off - a testament to the forces at work. I had barely escaped with my life. Over the next few weeks, I surfed very little and avoided bigger waves - because I now had a hell of a respect for them.

Semester abroad in Bali

I had already been in Bali for a while at that point. I was studying Intercultural Management at the university in Denpasar, the capital of the Indonesian island. For four months, I studied together with about 100 other German students study subjects such as Indonesian culture and history, business management case studies, international marketing and even Indonesian language.

It was chance that brought me here. I had actually wanted to study in Spain for a year and work towards a double degree as part of our university's partner program. To do this, you had to gain a certain number of credit points in a foreign language at one of the partner universities. I took Spanish courses at the UAS. But as my progress in Spanish was lagging behind that of my fellow students, I was worried that it would be quite difficult to study seriously in Spanish. I was far from fluent. When my fellow student Maren told me on the bus that she wanted to study in Bali next semester, my ears perked up. By the end of the bus ride, I had decided to apply for the Bali program as well and to scrap my plans for Spain.

Together with my fellow student Maren, I slowly got to know other people from the course who came from all over Germany. Most of them were studying sports or economics. We teamed up with Dax and Anne and rented a guesthouse in Kuta. We had nice, clean rooms there, all set around a pool. Everyone had their own little terrace, separated by lots of green plants - a touch of the jungle.

Even though we didn't become close friends straight away, it was a relief to have made my first connection. Because my symptoms and anxiety continued to make it difficult to make new acquaintances or friends.

We had lessons from Monday to Wednesday and initially traveled the route from Kuta to Denpasar together by cab. Everything cost very little and as a student you could afford a lot of luxuries. For example, we went out to eat two or three times a day. For five marks you could eat your fill with a pizza and a Coke or order a local rice dish for two marks. On Thursdays there were always excursions where we visited businesses or cultural institutions. Bali was the only island in the otherwise Muslim-dominated country to have a Hindu religious majority. You could see this everywhere in the exotic temples and the small spirit houses that were installed in front of many entrances to make small offerings to the spirits and gods. Small bowls of incense, juice and sweets were often placed on the street to appease the gods. These offerings were arranged several times a day and were part of daily religious customs.

In the meantime, I had made friends with the people from Mainz. They were a group of students, all but one of whom studied at Mainz University of Applied Sciences. Stefan, Karina, Simona and Karo were studying business administration. Danny had come along as Stefan's buddy and was studying industrial engineering in Mannheim. I was surprised that I somehow still managed to make friends. I went on lots of excursions with the people from Mainz. We visited temples, spent weekends together on the nearby Gili Islands, snorkeled and partied together in the discos in Kuta.

On the surface, I enjoyed a carefree time. I studied very little, had enough time and money to go on great excursions and found myself in a tropical paradise where everyone wanted to go on vacation. The air temperature was a constant 30 degrees and the water 29 degrees the whole time. You could wear shorts, a T-shirt and flip-flops every day without a second thought and were always dressed appropriately. We went to the beach almost every day to sunbathe or surf. It felt like a permanent vacation with short interruptions to pop into university.

For someone with chronic pain, even such a situation, however, is only the outer façade, while something completely different is going on inside. It was a paradox. My circumstances were just about as phenomenal as I could have wished for. But even when I was enjoying the outings with the Mainzern, I was constantly tormented by the pain in my head and neck. Sometimes it was so bad that I felt sick as a dog and would have preferred to be alone. But that was usually not possible on these outings and I had to bear it bravely. I then became even quieter than I already was.

In my current home, in the hotel room at Kedins Inn 2, I usually practiced progressive muscle relaxation once or twice a day for 30 minutes. This helped a little to reduce the tension and bring the pain level down a little. But on such trips, we often shared rooms and it was difficult to take this time, especially as I hadn't told the others about my complaints. I was still embarrassed by my condition. Who could understand that you were constantly and permanently accompanied by pain and that everything and every situation in life was affected by it? That it had developed into anxiety, panic attacks and depressive thoughts over time? I still didn't believe that being open about my illness would bring me any benefits. So I became a master at hiding my negative feelings, because I was sure that the intensity and permanence of these would also overwhelm those around me. I hid them in my laughter; I hid them in my silence; I hid them by saying I was fine, even though the opposite was true.

I felt best when I was drinking alcohol. With increasing alcohol levels, everything was much easier to bear. The alcohol numbed the pain, relaxed the muscles and reactivated my speech center to a certain extent. That's why I loved to party and I regularly drank a little more to get really intoxicated. These bouts of intoxication were like a little release, like a vacation from my permanent state of misery. These alcoholic outbursts gave me a certain kind of strength. I felt that deep down, there was still a version of me that was able to act in a freer state than I was used to in my everyday life.

I liked this person. I didn't like the person I had become without the alcohol at all. Nevertheless, I had a natural aversion to permanently drowning my miserable state in alcohol. It just seemed wrong to me. I drank two to three times a week.

I quickly fell in love with Karina from the Mainz clique. She had a great laugh, a beautiful, deep voice and a pretty face. She was rather reserved, but very self-confident in her own way. I really liked her, but I couldn't make advances or get close to her. I had too many blocks and fears inside me for that. Sometimes I tried to convince myself that I might have a chance with her. But I was basically sure that although she liked me as a buddy in the clique, I was out of the question for anything more. It was frustrating to see her every day but not be able to get as close to her as I would have liked. Because I had the feeling that she could have been interested in the earlier version of me.

At the end of the semester, she started dating another fellow student. That depressed me, because it seemed to rub my own inadequacy in my face. Would I ever have a girlfriend again?

Wherever I could overcome myself, however, I enthusiastically used my newly acquired language skills. After just two months, I was able to make small talk with the locals. The Bahasa Indonesia language was relatively easy to learn because it used the Latin writing system and was phonetically surprisingly similar to German pronunciation. It was an artificially introduced language in order to have a common language base among the many

Indonesian islands. Verbs were not conjugated and there were no tenses. Instead, one simply said „I swim today", "I swim yesterday". This meant you could use the language in everyday life in a relatively short time.

This was particularly helpful when haggling over prices on a daily basis. If you could negotiate in Indonesian, it was immediately clear that you were not a simple tourist and you were shown a certain form of respect. I enjoyed asking the Balinese about their living conditions and habits in order to learn more about the culture.

I also admired the way the locals lived their days. They didn't seem to worry much about the future. If they had money, they just spent it. Unlike the Germans, they didn't seem so ambitious. I got the impression that this was bad for the economy, but good for the general state of mind. The Balinese seemed remarkably balanced and cheerful to me. Many things didn't work as well as in Germany. For example, every time you ordered a large meal in a restaurant, you could be sure that the waiters would forget something or make a mistake. I always wondered why they didn't just write the order on a piece of paper. But that just didn't seem to be the norm. It worked that way too. Somehow everything worked - just like that.

Stagnation in the status quo

I also tried massages again in Bali. There was a massage parlor that offered special reflexology massage, which supposedly eliminated all kinds of ailments. So I thought to myself: why not try the Asian art of healing again? I booked a few sessions, even a one-hour session was unbeatably cheap at ten marks. However, it didn't really help. At least I felt a bit more relaxed than usual for an evening afterwards.

I was still taking the antidepressant amitriptyline, in high doses. As a result, I needed a lot of sleep, ten hours was normal. If nothing important was going on, I was very slow to wake up in the morning, and it could be up to twelve hours that I was more or less logged off. I also had a dry mouth from time to time. I was also only supposed to consume very small amounts of alcohol with this high medication. But I decided that the benefits of the alcohol more than outweighed the disadvantages of the potential side effects and hardly cared. I still didn't feel that this medication was doing me much good. But I felt that it could at least keep me at the status quo and prevent my situation from getting any worse. That's why I continued to take it, despite the side effects and reduced drive.

Fascination Bali

The best experience in Bali was a rafting tour through the jungle and rice fields. We had booked the tour a few days in advance and a minivan picked us up early in the morning at the Mainzers' bungalow complex. We drove for about two hours; first through Kuta, then further and further up into the mountains, deep into the jungle. Our small group split up into two rubber dinghies, so that there were three of us and one rubber dinghy guide each. This was necessary as the river had powerful rapids.

Our two guides had fun pulling each other into the water with their paddles. We all had great fun and got splashed here and there. At one point, our boat even capsized and we were glad that we had locked our valuables and cameras in a waterproof barrel. Impressive rock faces towered to the left and right, densely overgrown with all kinds of jungle plants. It was wonderful to immerse ourselves in this pristine wilderness, far away from the hustle and bustle of Kuta and the traders who constantly approached us to sell something.

When the monsoon really hit hard in December, there were times when brown brackish water stood up to 20 centimetres high in the streets and you had to wade through it in your flip-flops. Nobody left the house without an umbrella. At its peak, it rained almost continuously for six days and we couldn't do much. We spent most of the time sitting outside Stefan, Danny and Karina's bungalow and playing cards on the covered terrace. Stefan and Karina smoked a lot, and out of sheer boredom I took after them. So I stupidly started smoking cigarettes at the age of 21. I enjoyed that little flash you get from nicotine. It distracted me a little from the pain in the short term and was even better when combined with alcohol. I'd been smoking joints and bongs since I was 16, but until then I'd always kept my hands off normal cigarettes. Since I'd been in Bali, I'd only smoked a joint two or three times, otherwise it didn't come up and I didn't miss it. But the cigarettes were still a nice substitute.

By the end of the semester, we had suddenly all had enough of Bali and wanted to go somewhere else. The terrorist attacks of September 11, 2001 had changed the mood in the Muslim country. A war in Afghanistan seemed imminent, and it didn't really feel safe to travel outside Bali in the Muslim parts of Indonesia.

Once, when we went to the Gili Islands for a long weekend, we passed through the neighboring island of Lombok. As we were waiting for the ferry, a boy of about ten asked us in front of his friends: "Are you Americans?"

"We're from Germany," I replied.

The little boy then said: "You're lucky! If you were Americans, I'd shoot you!" He pointed his finger at me and imitated a firearm with his thumb.

It was just a little boy's prank, but it still gave us a fright. Because this episode gave us a good idea of the mood in the country. Americans were no longer welcome, at least among some of the population, and citizens of other Western countries were no longer quite so welcome either.

Many therefore traveled on to New Zealand or Australia after the semester. Most of them still had two months until the next semester in Germany would begin. I said goodbye to my friends and flew to Singapore first. I had rebooked this part of my return flight so that I could make a stopover in Thailand.

THE TURNING POINT - MONASTERY IN THAILAND

Destination Thailand

From the airport in Singapore, I took a cab to the bus station to travel from there to Bangkok by bus. The bus was due to leave about an hour later and took 24 hours to travel through Malaysia and the south and center of Thailand to Bangkok.

The bus looked modern and comfortable. The bus driver stowed our luggage down in the hold and I finally took my seat. A little later, a western-looking girl sat down in the seat next to me. She had long, curly hair and it turned out that she was from New Zealand. I liked her and we started talking about our travel plans. The interaction was exhausting as I was in a lot of pain, as usual. She told me about a friend who had taken part in a meditation course at a Buddhist monastery in Chiang Mai in northern Thailand. This immediately aroused my curiosity and, intrigued, I asked: "How long did the course last? What experiences did she have there? And what is the name of the monastery?" I wanted to know everything in detail.

But she replied: "I can't say for sure. In any case, my friend was very enthusiastic about the course. She found it through the tourist information office in Chiang Mai. I don't know any more than that."

At that very moment, I decided to travel to Chiang Mai after my upcoming vacation and look for this monastery and the meditation course there.

Vacation for three

As my next semester in Kiel wasn't due to start until two months later, I had arranged to go on a vacation to Thailand with my friends Ralle and Jens. We met in Bangkok, in a hotel on the infamous Khao San Road, a backpacker hotspot.

I enjoyed a great ten days in Thailand with my friends. We traveled from Bangkok to the south. We first spent two days on the island of Koh Samui and the remaining days on the neighboring island of Koh Phangan. There were lots of backpackers, dropouts and hippies on Koh Phangan, and we rented a beautiful hut right on the beach at Hat Rin. Our hut was built into the rocky hillside and perched on long wooden stilts above the bay. From the balustrade we had a wonderful view over the whole bay with its sandy beach, small restaurants and bars, all surrounded by palm trees. We smoked joints together, had a delicious meal in the small town and explored the hilly, heavily wooded island on two scooters. We treated ourselves to a Thai massage almost every day, as it only cost five marks for an hour.

Between Christmas and New Year, one of the legendary full moon parties took place on the beach. We celebrated with thousands of other people on the beach under the full moon. Every bar had their sound systems turned up full blast. People danced wildly to electronic music, goa trance or reggae. We got drunk on beer and Redbull, mixed with local Mekong whiskey, and let ourselves be carried away by the party atmosphere. Various fire artists performed tricks with their torches to the beat of the music. We partied until the next morning and chatted drunkenly with other backpackers from all over the world. There was a cheerful party atmosphere all over the beach and the ambience was fantastic.

In the Buddhist monastery

On New Year's Day, my friends traveled back home. I myself made my way to Chiang Mai a day later. The friendly woman at the tourist information office gave me the address of a monastery that offered meditation courses. Full of anticipation for this adventure and full of hope that the meditation course could help me with my pain, but also full of fear of the unknown, I didn't want to wait another hour. That same day, I organized a yellow songthaew - a kind of shared cab - to take me there.

I was greeted by a friendly young monk. "Sawadee Krap" said the young monk and gave me a friendly smile. I had never been to a Buddhist monastery before and had never met a Buddhist monk. I didn't really know how to behave and said shyly: "Hello, I would like to do a meditation course. I have three weeks to spare."

"A full course normally lasts 28 days. But it's also good to be here for three weeks," replied the monk.

He had a strong Thai accent, but I was amazed at how good his English was. At the same time, I was relieved that he was friendly and open and that everything seemed so uncomplicated.

"You can stay right here and I'll do the registration with you."

"I still have my things at the hotel and would like to come back tomorrow," I replied.

"Okay, see you tomorrow then," he said goodbye with a smile and left.

The next day, the same songthaew driver drove me to the temple again. Before I got out of the car,

I quickly swatted a feisty mosquito between my hands. My driver then burst out laughing and said: "You're a beautiful farang! I want to go meditate in the temple, but kill mosquitoes!" Farang is a Thai term for "stranger" or "Foreigners".

The saying stuck in my mind because my relationship with mosquitoes was to change over the next few weeks.

The young monk from the previous day took me in and completed the formalities with me. In the meantime, he made a few jokes and laughed a lot, which relaxed me a little. I was very excited - completely unaware of what I had actually got myself into and what life in a Buddhist temple like this might be like.

After he had taken my personal details, I was immediately given the first instructions on how to meditate. First of all, I was to sit on my knees on my heels and perform a mindful bow three times. I was to name the movements in my mind: "lifting, lifting, lifting, lowering, lowering, lowering" and so on. In general, I was to name everything I did in my mind - when walking, eating, thinking, seeing. He then showed me the walking meditation and the sitting meditation. I did the exercises after him and at the same time tried to name for myself what I was doing.

After the brief introduction, the monk took me to the wardrobe and dressed me in the white clothes that lay meditators traditionally wear. He then showed me to my room.

The next day, the same monk called me into the meditation hall and went through the meditation technique with me in more detail. He showed me the mindful bowing again in detail, then the walking meditation, followed by the sitting meditation. Each round of meditation went like this. The mindful bowing lasted three to five minutes, followed by ten minutes walking and ten minutes sitting. This corresponded to a round of meditation, after which I was supposed to take a 20-minute break before practicing the next round. And I was always supposed to name everything in my mind. You gave a mental label to the activity you were doing. For walking meditation, for example, I named 'right goes thus , left goes thus'. For sitting meditation, you named "rising-falling" and be aware of the movement of the abdominal wall. If thoughts arose, you should name them three times with "thinking, thinking, thinking" and then let them go. Also, if you became aware of emotions or sensations, you should name them and let them move again. I found the technique immediately appealing and plausible and had the feeling that I could easily get involved with it. I was very curious to see what would happen if I managed to observe myself at this extremely detailed level over a longer period of time.

During my time in the monastery, I lived in my own small kuti with my own bathroom. A kuti was a small house where monks and nuns usually lived, but also meditators who were visiting the monastery. My kuti was very simply furnished, with a bed, a chair and a small shelf. It was getting on in years and wasn't the cleanest, but I felt reasonably comfortable. At least I had my own space. Luckily I had brought my own mosquito net, because the mosquito screens on the windows had small holes in some places. So I didn't have to worry about malaria. There was a calm atmosphere in the temple. You couldn't say it was a huge monastery, but it wasn't exactly small either. There were various monastery buildings with golden decorations that blended in well with the numerous shady trees. A beautiful mixture of gold and green. There were about 30 lay meditators in the monastery, who could be recognized by their white clothing. There were around 30 to 40 monks and about the same number of nuns. The monks wore orange robes. The nuns, who were called Mae Chees, were also dressed in white robes, but unlike the lay meditators, they had their hair cut short like the monks. The monks and nuns also each lived in their own small kuti huts, which were located in separate areas.

Once a day, I had a short, five to ten-minute conversation with the abbot of the monastery. The head of the monastery assigned new meditation tasks and I was able to ask brief questions. On some days he increased my meditation time by five minutes, on other days he added something to the sequence of steps or the sitting meditation. When I had already been there for a few days, I was asked to perceive and name various points of contact on my body in sequence while sitting, alternating with my breathing and sitting position. However, naming seemed to be the most important thing. The abbot attached particular importance to this. Whenever I told him about my knee or back pain, I was asked the same question: "Did you label it?"

In principle, I was free to organize my daily routine as I wished. However, I was supposed to go to bed at 10 p.m., get up at 4 a.m. and practice meditation throughout the day, with 20-minute breaks between rounds. I could meditate alone in my own kuti or in the meditation hall with others. It was up to everyone.

I was extremely excited to see what meditating would do to me. I was secretly hoping for some kind of earthquake, a euphoric state of happiness or a deep trance in which I left my body and floated through the air. For the first two or three days, there were no major experiences. I simply tried to follow the instructions as best I could and get used to everyday life in the monastery.

At four o'clock in the morning, a loud gong woke me up. However, I had enormous problems getting up at four in the morning. Although I resolved every evening to get up the next morning with the gong on time and in a disciplined manner, I regularly discarded this intention. I often only managed to get out of bed at five or six o'clock, meditated for a short while and then went to breakfast. The mornings and evenings were quite chilly. I therefore bought a slightly thicker white sweater in the small monastery store. I was impressed by the Mae Chee, who was usually in charge of the monastery store, as she seemed to be in constant meditation. When she walked around somewhere, she walked very slowly and deliberately, looking intently at her feet. In the monastery store, she usually sat on her chair with her hands folded and her eyes closed. But when she was approached, she was immediately present, with alert eyes and kind features.

I had warm rice soup for breakfast every day at six in the morning. It didn't taste particularly good to me, but I could eat it and it served its purpose. As the meditation course took place in what is known as 'noble silence', no one talked while we ate and we were supposed to focus on eating. The monk had told me at the beginning that I should also name every little detail of the process while eating. For example, "seeing", "wanting", "taking", "touching", "chewing", "tasting", "sweet", "sour", "swallowing", "wanting" and so on. In general, I was supposed to mentally label everything I did during the day - whether I was drinking tea or going to the toilet.

The highlight of the day, lunch, took place every day at eleven o'clock. There were often rice dishes with various vegetables. You could also eat with meat, but I preferred to be careful because I'd had bad experiences in the past and didn't trust the cold chain when it came to meat. That's why I always joined the vegetarian queue. The food usually tasted quite good and I always put a large amount on my plate as there was no other meal for the rest of the day. After 12 noon, you were only allowed to eat dairy-based food, which meant buying warm soy milk from a stall outside the monastery for a few Thai baht in the evening. I managed quite well with that; I had something warm in my stomach and I didn't get too hungry. The more days I spent there, the better I got used to it.

A silver lining on the horizon

On the fourth day, I finally noticed some changes in my perception. As I was tying my shoes, I noticed that I was absolutely present and extraordinarily aware of the tying process. I was completely free of thoughts for a few moments and lost myself completely in this activity. Everything else in the world was not important, not relevant at that moment. The only thing that mattered was tying my shoes, and this moment gave me absolute satisfaction. It was perfect. I thought, "Wow, life can be that simple!"

It was also on this day that my perception of taste and all other sensory perceptions began to intensify and everything looked more beautiful, shiny and special than usual. I found myself simply looking at the leaves of a tree for five minutes in fascination. It was as if I had really seen leaves for the first time in my life. As if I had never really noticed them before because it was always so loud in my head. Fascinated, I walked through the monastery in the evening and enjoyed all the beautiful sights of the golden Buddhas in the dim light. It was a bit like having a weed - except you're not so crazy but, on the contrary, was extremely clear-headed.

After a few meditations, I felt calm, clear and peaceful, a bit like being reborn. For the first time in years, I felt a peace and joy within me that I had thought was almost gone forever. I now also felt a tender hope budding within me that this kind of meditation could help me with my chronic pain. It seemed to me that the pain impulse was still there constantly. But the meditation process changed the perception of the painful feeling in some mysterious way which made me more detached from it. And that had a positive effect.

I realized that three weeks of meditation would probably not cure me. But I had the feeling that I might be able to retrain my pain memory with years of intensive practice. First of all, however, I was really happy that after years of pain, after years of ever worsening complaints, after years in which I had tried countless unsuccessful and frustrating therapies, I had finally found a working weapon in the fight against pain. At last I was no longer completely helpless at its mercy, but could actively do something to improve my condition.

In the meditation hall, I carefully observed the other meditators. Western-looking foreigners as well as Thais were practising here. Many practiced walking meditation at a different pace to me and I assumed that they had already progressed further in the course. I was particularly impressed by one meditator who practiced one hour of walking meditation and one hour of sitting meditation. He was probably in his early thirties and looked East Asian. His sitting position looked very disciplined and professional. After a while, his upper body began to sway back and forth relatively quickly. It made a big impression on me, because it looked as if this movement came from an enormous amount of excess energy, which caused his upper body to sway. It was clear to me that this must be an extremely advanced yogi with great meditative skills.

There were also some Thai women. They even liked to chat a bit during the day and, strictly speaking, did not really adhere to the Noble Silence. Nevertheless, their evening meditation seemed to work better than mine. In sitting meditation, they rocked back and forth very slowly and gently. It looked very graceful and I was convinced that these women had also reached a deep meditative state. I was a little annoyed that they managed to do this despite their daily conversations, while I was much more disciplined and probably still a long way from such deep states.

Over the next few weeks, I reflected a lot on my previous life while meditating. I realized how limited and painful it had been over the last few years. I imagined what would improve now and what it might look like in a few months or years. Labeling things became easier over time and I managed to label more and more things, whether it was the opening of a door or an emotion or sensory perception. Nevertheless, I still often drifted off in my thoughts during walking and sitting meditation and sometimes only noticed it late, after ten seconds, after 30 seconds, sometimes only after five or ten minutes. During sitting meditation, I had a lot of problems with my knees when sitting for long periods. I found it difficult to sit cross-legged and had pain, so I often stopped the session after 20 or 30 minutes. After three weeks of the meditation course, I had managed to do 40 minutes of walking and 40 minutes of sitting with iron discipline, but it remained a mystery to me how I was supposed to keep it up for an hour. Unfortunately, I couldn't finish the course, which actually lasted 28 days. Katrin, a friend of mine, came to Thailand to visit. I had to go back to Bangkok to receive her. Although I wasn't able to complete the course, the Meditating left a deep, lasting impression. It opened up a whole new dimension for me and gave me new hope that it would help me with the pain. Maybe my life would change now. Maybe one day I would be released from the prison of pain. From then on, I meditated every day. And after each meditation I felt the positive, liberating effect.

THE COMET IMPACT - MEDITATION COURSE IN BAVARIA

First changes

A few months after the meditation course in Thailand, there were some improvements in my life. I meditated every day for at least two hours. As I still had enough time in addition to my studies and it helped me a lot to cope with my everyday life and the pain, I often meditated for three or four hours a day. And I meditated at every opportunity: on the bus, in the waiting room at the doctor's, when climbing stairs or walking to the bus stop, I practiced mindful walking. I tried to label everything in everyday life as well as possible, from simple physical actions to emotions. Labeling was particularly easy with strong feelings of anger and anxiety. Due to their intensity, labeling them came automatically. This helped me a lot, especially in such charged situations, so that I didn't get caught up even deeper in these states - although I still had the feeling that I was at the mercy of my fear.

After meditating, I had significantly less pain, fewer worries and less anxiety for a while. I was able to express myself more clearly, was more optimistic and my everyday life became easier. Unfortunately, the main effect fizzled out quite quickly, after a few hours or so. By the time I had slept one night at the latest, it had largely disappeared again.

Nevertheless, the fact that I had found something at all that helped me and worked from the inside out gave me new courage, a new perspective and a new attitude to life. I still felt mentally locked up in my prison, but my cell was getting bigger and bigger

slowly with a little more exercise and comfort. I now had hope that one day I might even be able to leave prison.

This perspective also gave me new freedom in my everyday life and the feeling that I was no longer at the mercy of everything. Even though I spent an enormous amount of time meditating, it seemed more valuable to me, for example, to spend just one hour with friends in a contented, happy state than - without meditation - to have more time together but not be able to enjoy it because of the pain and negative emotions and only be able to act to a limited extent anyway.

The foundations of mindfulness

During my stay in a monastery in Thailand, a German nun who lived there gave me a flyer from a German meditation teacher in Bavaria. Her name was Hildegard Huber. I contacted her and signed up for a meditation course in

August 2002, which took place in a Bavarian Benedictine monastery - a good four months after my return from Asia.

I got on the train in Hamburg early in the morning and traveled all day. I had to change trains twice and finally took a cab at my destination station to take me to the monastery. I was probably too late, because at first I couldn't find anyone in the arrivals area of the monastery. However, a few kitchen utensils and half-unpacked boxes indicated that the course must be taking place here somewhere.

I wandered through the huge, imposing Benedictine monastery with its thick walls and finally came across an Asian-looking man with a camera around his neck on a staircase. I asked him: "Hello, is there a meditation course going on here somewhere?"

He laughed and patted me on the shoulder. "Come, come."
he said. I followed him up the stairs to a function room on the top floor, where about 30 people dressed in white were already sitting on the floor.

The opening ceremony of the meditation course began immediately. It turned out that the Asian-looking man was called Thanat and was Hildegard's meditation teacher, who had traveled all the way from Thailand to teach. Thanat sat cross-legged next to Hildegard in front of the group. After a friendly greeting, he thanked Hildegard and other helpers for organizing the course. I had some trouble understanding his English as he seemed to speak with a Thai accent. I estimated him to be in his late 50's. He made a dynamic, confident and humorous impression and incorporated all kinds of jokes into his explanations, often bursting into infectious laughter himself.

There was a Buddha statue at the front of the room, with four plates in front of it. The first plate was decorated with five flowers, five candles and five incense sticks. There were only two flowers, candles and incense sticks on each of the other plates. Thanat explained that the plates represented different aspects of the Dhamma, the Buddha's teachings, and that the ceremony was important to develop a good foundation and mindset for meditation practice.

The first plate stood for the respect and appreciation of Buddha, Dhamma, Sangha (community), parents and teachers and meditation practice.

The second plate stood for the eight rules of virtue that one tried to observe during a meditation course or retreat.

The third plate stood for the request to the teacher to receive instruction in meditation practice.

Finally, the fourth plate was about students and teachers asking each other in advance for forgiveness for any transgressions and violations that may have occurred during the course in thought, speech or action. This was intended to create a peaceful atmosphere for the course.

Each plate was held against the Buddha statue for a brief moment by one or more meditators after three bows. This was followed by various Pali recitations, which we repeated after Hildegard. I had already learned in the monastery that Pali was an ancient written language that had prevailed during the early spread of Buddhism and in which most of the texts of Theravada Buddhism were recorded.

After the ceremony, Thanat explained the basics of Vipassana meditation. "Vipassana"was introduced with "Insight meditation" translated. It means seeing things as they are. It is also said: „to see the true nature of things".

The teacher then explained the four foundations of mindfulness: body, feelings, mind and mind objects.

Mindfulness and labeling are practiced and trained in these four areas. We should observe and label which of the four main body positions we are currently in: sitting, standing, walking or lying down. We should also label smaller movements of the body, such as stretching, standing up and turning. Raising and lowering the abdominal wall and labeling the steps during walking meditation were also part of mindfulness for the body.

Then we should be mindful of feelings, whereby feelings were understood differently from what is generally accepted in the West. There were three types of feelings: positive, negative and neutral. We should also become aware of these by labeling them. For example, by labeling them with "pleasant, pleasant, pleasant" or "unpleasant, unpleasant, unpleasant" or "neutral, neutral, neutral".

We should train mindfulness of the mind by observing the thoughts and naming them, for example, "think, think, think" or "plan, plan, plan". We should then let go of the thoughts and stop pursuing the current topic.

Mental objects include all emotions that we should also name, for example "Fear, fear,

fear", "worry, worry, worry", and so on. Furthermore, mind objects also include all sensory perceptions experienced through the five senses. For example, if we heard a loud noise during walking meditation, we should stop and say "hear, hear, hear".

During the course, we also practiced observing the eight Buddhist precepts. These rules were as followed:

1. Do not harm any living creatures, for example flies or mosquitoes.

2. No lying and no thoughtless speech such as blasphemy or swearing. During the course, we practiced Noble Silence and spoke only when necessary.

3. Do not steal and do not take what has not been given.

4. Do not practice any sexual acts.

5. Do not consume drugs or alcohol.

6. Avoiding any form of entertainment or embellishment. This included activities such as singing, dancing, reading, internet, but also wearing perfume and jewelry.

7. No solid foods should be eaten after noon. Milk-based foods such as yogurt or chocolate without nuts and fruit were okay.

8. And we were supposed to sleep less, we only slept for six hours.

The course taught the same meditation technique with walking and sitting meditation as well as labeling, which I already knew from the monastery in Thailand. The method was taught in the tradition of the venerable Ajahn Tong Sirimangalo, who was a highly respected meditation teacher and abbot of a meditation monastery in Thailand. And of course the course also took place in Noble Silence. Hildegard taught the meditation students together with Thanat.

We only spoke during the daily reports with the teacher. Thanat, Hildegard and two or three other people sat in the reporting room as assessors. It seemed as if they were sitting there in a kind of training role. So I came into this room and it felt like I was being called into a doctor's office or for interrogation. The reportings scared the hell out of me because I hated being the center of attention and exposing myself to several pairs of eyes. After all, I wasn't here to have a good time or to have interesting experiences, but because I had serious physical and psychological problems and hoped that meditating would solve them.

Talking about it in front of several people was pretty much the worst thing I could imagine. When I sat in the waiting line in front of the reporting room, I regularly got palpitations and even panic attacks. When I did go in, I was barely able to speak sensible sentences, let alone describe my meditation experiences in a meaningful way.

I made an effort to hide my anxious state from the others. At least I was able to use the meditation technique and deal with these situations with labeling "Panic, panic, panic" or "fear, fear, fear". However, my acceptance of these conditions was limited. I hated the panic, and I hated the fear because it made my life so miserable. But I realized that labeling had a certain calming effect. Sometimes it actually eased or even stopped the spiral of anxiety that was building up.

I was given new tasks and exercises every day, and Thanat asked very strange questions: "Is there an itch somewhere, maybe ants crawling on your arm? Do you see disgusting pictures, dead people perhaps?"

I couldn't do anything with the questions at first. I found them very strange and tried to answer them as best I could.

to answer with "yes" and "no". In the end, I was simply relieved when I could leave the room again and had completed the daily reporting session for the day.

As I already had some practice, I started with 20 minutes, and every day the teacher increased my walking and sitting meditation by another five minutes. This time my knees didn't give me as much trouble as they had during the last course in Thailand. After nine days, I even managed to practise one hour of walking meditation and one hour of sitting meditation. I was extremely proud and satisfied that I actually managed to sit for an hour.

After a few days, I was also supposed to do metta meditation after sitting meditation. This involved sending good wishes and thoughts to myself in my mind, and then to other people such as family or friends. Finally, I was to extend these good wishes to all living beings. This spoke as follows: "May I be free from sorrow and pain, free from greed, hatred and delusion and protected from all dangers. May I live contentedly and happily. May my mom, dad, brothers and sister and all my other relatives, friends and acquaintances be free from grief and sorrow, free from greed, hatred and delusion, may they be protected from danger and may they live contented and happy."

I found it a bit strange and artificial at first to send out these wishes. Sometimes I also felt so full of negative feelings that it seemed absurd to speak them. But over time and with regular repetition, I began to like it. I imagined that a positive feeling arose when sending the metta. I now practiced this metta meditation for a few minutes after each sitting meditation.

Before going to bed, I should now also practise sleep meditation. When I go to bed, I should label everything mindfully and then observe the lifting and lowering of the abdominal wall in my normal sleeping position and label it "rising, falling". Thanat said: "Don't concentrate so much on the movement. It's just about being aware of the rising and falling. If you focus too much, you might not fall asleep."

After this remark, he burst into a loud, infectious laugh, which I found very likeable. It came out in almost all the reports, sometimes more, sometimes less. Then - just as suddenly as the laughter had started - he became more serious again: "You keep labeling until you fall asleep. And when you wake up the next morning, you start labeling again."

Smiling mischievously, he added: "If you are very mindful, you can tell the next morning whether you wake up with arise or a fall. Then label how you feel and also when you brush your teeth, shower and do other everyday tasks. Being mindful and labeling throughout the day supports your meditation practice."

Thanat asked me a few times when I had taken a seat on the cushion in the reporting room whether I had mindfully labeled opening the door and sitting down. I hadn't, of course, and he sent me out of the room so that I could do it again with mindfulness and labeling. Then he said: "You can move at a normal speed, otherwise strangers might think you're a bit weird." He started laughing again, and I joined in the laughter with a grin. "But the important thing is that you label it. It's like a book that you read over and over again. At some point, you know the whole text by heart and it's really easy."

The power of emotions

This meditation course was very different to the course in Thailand. The meditation instructions were explained in more detail, perhaps also because of the much more proportionate teacher-student ratio. I also no longer had as much pain in my knees and was able to do the longer sitting meditations better. As far as sleep was concerned, I naturally didn't manage to work out whether I woke up with a rising or a falling. I tried as hard as I could not to exceed the required six hours of sleep. However, I only managed this sometimes, as I was still taking the amitriptyline. I concealed my medication when I filled out the registration form. I also didn't tell anyone about it during the course as I was afraid that I might not be allowed to take part. I was also still deeply ashamed of it.

I felt much more emotionally upset during this retreat. I regularly had severe panic attacks and anxiety. Sometimes, however, joyful and positive, even ecstatic feelings and thoughts would arise during the meditation sessions, unleashing my curiosity about what was to come. But in the end, I had no idea what to expect. The teacher's questions got weirder and weirder, my emotional explosions became more and more intense. I hid my panic attacks and anxiety from the teacher, even in the reports, because I was afraid I wouldn't be allowed to continue. And I really wanted to carry on! I intuitively felt that I was on the right path, even though I felt like I was in a small nutshell on a stormy sea when it came to my emotions.

The pain changed during the course. It changed from a purely physical experience of pain to a more vibrational, energetic experience of pressure, hardness, tightness and generally negative energy. This was in the neck area, in the temples, in the whole head, but also down to between the shoulder blades. The whole area felt like pressure and tightness. However, it was very different from the classic pain experience that I felt in everyday life. Nevertheless, this experience also often produced very unpleasant and negative feelings. The longer the course lasted, the more intense everything felt. The meditations became deeper and the perception of energy and pulsation increased.

Often the whole negative intensity overwhelmed me so much that the meditation sessions ended in frustration. Again and again my attention was drawn to the area in my neck that felt uncomfortable, hard and stiff, and I often couldn't get it away. It was as if a huge magnet was pulling my attention with force. When I tried to draw it back to my breath, I was relatively unsuccessful. I was unsure whether I was meditating incorrectly. 'This can't be right,' I doubted. I then went to Thanat or the reporting room several times and tried to discuss it. I explained my concerns as best I could and then Thanat asked questions:

"During walking meditation, do you concentrate on the movement of the foot or are you aware of the movement?"

What kind of strange question was that again? At first I

didn't really know where he was going with it.

"What do you mean?" I asked.

"Where is your mind? Is it by the foot or is it somewhere else?" Thanat asked back.

"Yes, my mind is on the foot." I still didn't really know what he meant.

"You can't focus on the movement. That's too intense, too much concentration, too much focus. Make it simpler, just be aware of the movement. That is mindfulness. Mindfulness is like water, concentration is like fire. You need more water, less fire," he explained.

First of all, I thought I understood to some extent what he was getting at. At first, I thought my concerns had been resolved. But a few hours later I had the feeling again that I was doing something wrong and asked again the next day. After all, I wanted to do everything right if I was already here and meditating for countless hours a day. Hildegard also tried to give me more explanations and clarify my questions. She always had good answers, but when I meditated on my own again, I wondered whether I was really doing everything right.

Apart from these irritations, meditating worked quite well on the whole.

Insights, doubts, happiness and liberation

The more I meditated, the more I realized that the pain, the panic attacks, the fear, the negative thoughts and this feeling of pressure in the whole upper body were all connected. All these phenomena had become tangled up in each other like a ball of wool and were influencing each other. After my pain had become chronic, it had become an illness in its own right. As a result, I was no longer able to do many of the things I would have liked to do in my life, or I failed to do them. Every negative situation I had experienced since then had created new negative feelings and frustration, and these accumulated in this "tangled ball of mud" and were stored there. With each new negative experience, the tangle became even more powerful and enormous. I then subconsciously associated these negative experiences with the pain in my neck, which became even more powerful and attracted negative vibrations and stored them in my body. So that's how the pain memory worked! If it can be programmed like this, I thought, then it must also be be possible to reverse this effect through meditation. I started to believe in it.

Towards the end of the course, the negative states of panic and anxiety, grueling self-doubt and feeling of pressure in my neck became so great and overwhelming that I decided to end the course prematurely before I possibly developed psychosis or something similar. I went to Thanat and told him about it:

"Thanat, I have severe anxiety and pain. It's all so intense! Far too intense! I'm afraid I'm going crazy. I think it's better if I stop the course now."

Thanat listened to me attentively, but didn't seem particularly impressed by the descriptions of my personal hell.

"Where is the pain?" he asked.

"It's worst in the neck, and then it goes up into my head and temples," I replied.

He replied calmly but firmly: "Sit on the sofa there in a meditation position. Until I say 'stop', focus your attention for a few minutes on the spot in your neck where it hurts. And just stay with that spot."

I did as he said. As I had been meditating for many days and hours in the meantime, my perception was very fine and everything was very intense. Focusing on the spot on the back of my neck also felt very intense. Thanat sat quietly next to me and said after a few minutes: "Just keep going until I say stop".

I don't know exactly how long it took. Maybe after 10 to 15 minutes, Thanat said: "Okay, you can slowly open your eyes now. How do you feel now?"

I tried to assess my condition. I noticed that the pressure in my neck had eased considerably, that I felt calmer overall and no longer felt panicky. "I feel better, the pressure in my neck has eased a little, I said."

Thanat grinned at first and then laughed heartily: "You see, don't worry and go back to meditating. You'll get through it in one piece! After the course, I'll show you a special exercise that will help you with your pain." Relieved, I went back to my room and marveled at what had happened. I had so much faith in Thanat that I was almost no longer worried that something bad could happen to me. I felt that Thanat exuded the competence and authority needed to teach this extremely intense meditation technique. I was convinced that he knew what he was doing. It was probably just that my states of mind bordering on madness were a regular part of the 'process' and that everything would turn out well in the end.

In the last intensive phase of the meditation retreat, amazing things happened that completely shook me to my core and were difficult to describe in words.

I was sitting cross-legged in sitting meditation and a kind of tension built up in my body, which was released as if by magic in a sudden, violent twitch. My head jerked to the left or right with a loud, internal cracking sound. The cracking sound was similar to the sound you hear when a chiropractor adjusts your body. However, I didn't think anyone other than me could have heard it. It was more on an internal, energetic level. Immediately afterwards, I felt relieved, as if I had just shed the ballast that I had been carrying around with me for many years. It was umpteen times better than an orgasm! My head became clearer and more alert, I felt more and more in the present moment. I realized that thinking was thinking, seeing was seeing, feeling was feeling and that all perceptions were linked to ideas, opinions, associations and emotions. I also understood that these were constantly developing and influencing each moment in the unconscious.

I became more and more aware of my conditioning through meditation.

These jerks occurred spontaneously a few hundred times. Some were rather small and somewhat pleasant. Others had a greater force and intensity, and immediately afterwards I felt a strong sense of elation and greater alertness. I felt reborn, as if I was breaking my way out of my mental prison with each of these convulsions! This experience made me tremble with awe.

Everything I experienced in this meditation course left a lasting impression on me. The experiences reminded me of Pavlov's principle, which we had studied in ninth grade biology class. In a scientific experiment, a dog was presented with food and a bell was rung at the same time. In anticipation of the food, the dog produced more saliva. This process was repeated several days in a row. Finally, the dog was no longer given food, but only the bell was rung. This time, too, the dog produced more saliva. The dog was now conditioned to the bell and subconsciously associated the bell with feeding.

In principle, this conditioning process works in the same way in humans. For example, I was conditioned to increase my neck tension in unpleasant situations when I had to give a presentation or was otherwise the center of attention. As the tension increased, so did nervousness, anxiety and panic. These negative feelings caused the tension to increase even further and in turn intensified the negative feelings This went on and on - no matter how much I tried to stay calm, I couldn't control it. Deep in my subconscious, the behavioral patterns were conditioned in such a way that I reacted with tension, fear and panic in certain situations. In contrast, I was completely powerless. Neither rational thought nor enormous willpower could change these patterns of behavior. They were set in stone and I felt powerless to change them.

During the two-week meditation course, I realized how this conditioning actually took place, step by step. In a certain situation, memories of similar past situations were automatically recalled. As these previous situations had been negative, with a lot of uncertainty and fear, negative thoughts developed, which caused negative feelings and physical sensations such as tension in the neck. These negative feelings and physical sensations in turn evoked negative memories. It was like an infinite spiral, and all this negativity became linked and conditioned through the sensation of tension in the neck. The tension in turn evoked thoughts and memories that were heavily laden with negative emotions such as aversion, fear and panic. In meditation, I was able to observe this chain of reactions in 'real time'. In part, I had already known about this beforehand - but not how I could do anything about it. I seemed to be powerless against this chain of reactions.

But now I learned how I could slowly undo this conditioning by labeling the individual parts of this reaction chain as they emerged. However, such behavioral patterns were stored deep in the subconscious. In order to achieve deconditioning, you had to penetrate deep levels of the subconscious. I suspected that this would only work with very intensive meditation over many days.

At the end of the course, Thanat explained to the participants, who were doing a course like this for the first time, which stages you went through in such a meditation course. In Vipassana meditation, there were so-called yanas, also known as stages of insight, which you went through during the course. At each stage, there were characteristic experiences that each meditator went through to a greater or lesser extent.

That explained a lot. It made it much easier for me to understand what I had experienced on the course. Now the strange questions that Thanat had often asked during the reports made a bit more sense to me.

The new attitude to life

After the drastic experience of the meditation course in the Bavarian monastery, I rarely experienced panic attacks in my everyday life. When they did occur, they were no longer as intense as they had been before. I had the feeling that I could manage it, for example by preparing extremely intensively for a lecture and practically memorizing it. This fact alone gave me much more confidence in my everyday life. As I used to get into situations several times a week that triggered panic attacks with a racing heart, this alone was nothing short of a miracle!

The headaches had reduced by a third since the course, and my hope that my life would now be much better again had increased. Even my omnipresent fears were no longer quite so massive and immovable. My self-confidence, which had been almost completely eroded over the last few years, grew a little again like a young, tender plant.

Since the basic course, I understood and felt myself to be a Buddhist and now believed in rebirth and karma. In meditation, I experienced how powerful the mind was and the tremendous force behind it. I could not imagine that it simply dissolved when the body no longer functioned adequately.

Retreat in Frankfurt

A lot had changed for the better in my life since the basic course. I was more optimistic. There were more and more phases in which I felt reasonably good and free. Nevertheless, there were still far too many negative situations, fears, pain and a feeling of powerlessness.

Six months later, I felt the desire to take another meditation course. I wanted to shed even more of this negative baggage. I hoped to further reduce my pain and gain even more of the freedom that I had regained since the last course.

Once you had completed the 15-day basic course, you could take part in ten-day retreats. I called Hildegard to find out whether there was an opportunity to do a retreat like this somewhere in Germany. She had given me the contact details of a Buddhist monastery in Frankfurt. There lived an Israeli Buddhist monk, Phra Ofer, who led Vipassana retreats. I called there and arranged a period in which I wanted to do the retreat in the small monastery.

The monastery was located in a normal house in the Götzenhain district of Frankfurt. Two Thai monks and Phra Ofer lived there. Every day they chanted together in the mornings and evenings, and Thai people often came by at lunchtime to bring food and offer it to the monks. At first I was the only one meditating. A few days later, another woman joined me. Every day I had a report with Phra Ofer. He asked me questions and explained more about what was happening in the retreat and what exactly I was experiencing.

In principle, the retreat was similar to the basic course, but condensed into ten days. However, as I already knew the technique in principle and was now able to had an idea of the process, I found it easier to switch from everyday study life to everyday meditation than last time. As I was the only one meditating at the beginning, there were virtually no distractions and I was able to concentrate fully on meditating.

While I had not learned much about the stages of insight in the basic course, I was initiated a little more into these stages of the meditation process in the retreat. Phra Ofer also told me about other Buddhist concepts.

He explained to me the three characteristics of existence - impermanence, suffering and non-self - which were particularly important in Buddhism and in meditation practice. Everything was subordinate to impermanence, so it had a beginning and an end. However, the fact that we as humans often clung to impermanent things resulted in suffering, for example. If you lost a loved one, that was suffering. If you fell ill, that was suffering. But it was also suffering when you wanted something and couldn't get it. For example, I wanted to have a girlfriend for years, but it just didn't work out, no matter how hard I tried. Not-self referred to not being able to control everything. Sometimes you wanted to meditate, but tiredness made it very difficult. Sometimes you wanted to be relaxed and calm, but you couldn't because you were so excited.

He also initiated me into the four noble truths proclaimed by the Buddha:

1. Every living being has experienced suffering in its life.
2. There are causes for this suffering.
3. These causes can been overcome.
4. The means by which this suffering could be overcome was the noble eightfold path.

The noble eightfold path was like the four noble truths of

of central importance in Buddhism:

1. Right view
2. Right thoughts
3. Right speech
4. Right action
5. Right livelihood
6. Right effort
7. Right concentration
8. Right mindfulness

He described the difference between concentration and mindfulness in an extremely humorous and lively way, as well as many other things. I had already read a few books about Vipassana and Buddhism in the months since the basic course. Together with the monk's explanations, I slowly gained a better insight into what the Buddhist teachings were about and what role meditation played in this:

In Theravada Buddhism, which is mainly practiced in Thailand, Myanmar and Sri Lanka, the goal is to end suffering and exit the cycle of existence by attaining Nibbana (Pali version of Nirvana). Three factors are important to enter the path of liberation: Ethics (sila), meditation (samadhi) and wisdom (panna). Only when these three factors are trained and cultivated is it possible to progress on the path of liberation.

In the area of ethics, there are the five precepts for normal everyday life and the extended eight precepts that should be observed during monastic stays or retreats. In principle, one should avoid bad deeds and, if possible, do good deeds. Bad deeds create bad karma, good deeds create good karma, whereby karma usually refers to effects in future lives. In addition, it is also important to show generosity or practicing generosity (dana). This teaches you to open your heart and let go. The monks and nuns in Thailand have dedicated their lives to the Dhamma, the teachings of the Buddha. They give discourses, lessons and instructions to anyone who wants to learn about it. As these are considered so valuable that they cannot be paid for in money, they are given according to the dana principle. In return, the lay followers in Thailand provide for the livelihood of the monks and nuns. Generosity is a quality of the mind that can be trained. It is essential for progress on the path and generates good karma.

In meditation, you train an your mind and free it from defilements (kilesas). These defilements include negative emotional patterns such as greed, fear and anger, as well as ignorance.

Wisdom is the result of an ethical lifestyle and meditative development. With increasing wisdom, ignorance decreases and one develops a deeper understanding of the interplay between body and mind.

While ethics is important in order not to create new, negative karma, but instead new, positive karma, old, negative karma can be dissolved through meditation.

In contrast to Theravada Buddhism, the goal in Mahayana Buddhism, which is practiced in Tibet and Japan, for example, is not one's own enlightenment and attainment of Nibbana. Instead, the aim is to become a perfect Buddha and remain in the cycle of existence and be reborn again and again until all living beings are liberated.

The house next door to the monastery in Frankfurt had a barn. The mice probably migrated from there. As monks do not harm living creatures however, they did not set any mousetraps - or only those with which they could catch them alive. This led to a peaceful coexistence of mice and monks in the house. There was also a mouse in my room. At first I was afraid it would nibble at me or crawl into my clothes while I was practicing sitting meditation. At first I found it difficult to meditate with a mouse in the room. But the more days went by, the more I became friends with her. I regularly sent her metta, loving kindness, and at some point I hardly minded her keeping me company. That's when I felt the power of sending metta.

Towards the end of the course, I experienced a longer phase in which the neck pain and negative emotions increased and I struggled with extreme states of anger. I kept stopping during the walking meditation, calling out "anger, anger, anger" and asking myself whether what I was doing could actually still be called meditation.

At some point after that, my heart started to twinge. It felt as if someone was stabbing me directly in the heart with a large knife. I instinctively grabbed my heart with both hands when the stabs came, sometimes I even bent my knees or doubled over a little. I got a fright because of the intensity and worried that I might have a heart attack. However, I was not completely unfamiliar with heart palpitations. I knew it from the past. I had had it for a few months in my early teens. At the time, the GP told me it was a growth phenomenon and would go away, which it did.

At the next reporting, I worriedly told Phra Ofer about my heartache. He laughed delightedly and said "Very good! That's a good sign and means that the mind is clearing! Don't worry about it. But if it comes back label it."

I was reassured by his answer, and when the stinging the next time it came, I called it "stinging, stinging, stinging". Because I now assumed that it was part of the cleansing process and was actually a good sign, I was no longer afraid. I was even a little pleased that the meditation seemed to be having an effect, and in a different way to the basic course.

I also experienced the twitching and tossing of the head that I was already familiar with from the basic course, but this time not nearly as often and not as intensively as in the first course.

The last few days of the retreat didn't go as well for me as the first course. I didn't feel as awake and clear, instead there was a lot of negativity. The overwhelming feeling of peace and relief that I had felt last time was also largely absent. Maybe I had done something wrong? However, I had no idea what it could have been. I did have the feeling that I had learned and cleansed a lot. But it didn't feel like it had reduced my pain by another 30 percent; more like another three to four percent.

During this retreat, however, my fears did not come to the fore as much. Although I had a few minor phases of paranoia during the course, there were no major anxiety attacks. Instead, I had to deal more with angry states. Nevertheless, I was curious to see whether I would notice a change in my everyday life afterwards.

MAIN STUDY PROGRAM - ON THE PATH OF COMPUTER SCIENCE AND MEDITATION

Meditation in everyday life

In the months and years that followed, I meditated a lot in my everyday life and went on a ten-day retreat about once a year. My pain, as well as my fears and feelings of inferiority, became a little less with each retreat. Practicing helped me to cope better with everyday life and to better control my sometimes extremely negative emotions in problematic situations. It helped me not to take out my anger and frustration on other people, and I no longer fed my negative behavior patterns with so much new negative energy. After meditating, I always felt more optimistic, more energetic and more eager to meet and interact with other people.

Business informatics

I specialized in business informatics in my main degree course in business administration. Many of my fellow students chose two main subjects in order to have better chances on the job market later on. I didn't want to overextend myself and thought it was better to concentrate on one major. I liked my new subjects such as SAP, Information Management and Software Engineering. I found it easier to study now, as I had fewer hours than in the foundation course and the IT subjects interested me much more than many of the business subjects I had previously had to take. I also attended lectures and courses at the Department of Computer Science in C++ programming, Java programming and databases to deepen my IT knowledge.

As I was now living on the west bank near the bigger university in a student residence, I had to travel 45 minutes by bus to the east bank, where the university og applied sciences was located. I used the journey time to meditate and study. I often read my Java programming book, a 1000-page tome that my parents had given me for Christmas.

Even now, I still found it difficult to make real contacts with my fellow students. I still had problems communicating and expressing myself, and sometimes I still stuttered a little. I was still a long way from the skills I once had before the pain came into my life.

Fortunately, I still benefited in this respect from my wild youth, in which I had built up a large circle of friends and many acquaintances. Surprisingly, many connections still existed. There were regular reunions with old acquaintances that I had known for many years. Many of them had also come to Kiel to study, or we saw each other when I visited my old home.

Konrad and Suse had chosen different majors for their main studies, which is why I saw them less and less. They also both had double majors and therefore spent a lot of time studying. Nevertheless, the time didn't get too long for me; at least I was able to get enthusiastic about the subject matter and I used the increased free time to meditate. I continued to do this every day for at least two hours, and on some days even longer.

If I wanted to do something with friends, I always planned it so that I had at least an hour and a half to meditate beforehand. That reduced my pain level and I felt much more unrestricted in my thoughts, speech and actions. If I also consumed alcohol in this state, I could really enjoy the time with my friends. At least on some of these evenings, I felt really good.

Even if these brief phases of cheerful exuberance with

one and a half hours of meditation preparation and a lot of alcohol, they still gave me a lot of hope and strength. After all, I had sorely missed the joy of simply being carefree and exuberant for many years. Relationships with my old friends also slowly improved and became closer again.

New in the student residence

There were five of us living in my hall of residence. We each had a twelve square meter room to ourselves, and we shared a large common room and a small kitchen.

Aron moved in shortly after me. He studied literature and a minor in musicology. He was even shyer and more reserved than me, a sensitive artistic soul. He brought a violin and a Playstation with him and regularly put us through our paces with his violin playing. Even as I was the opposite of a classical music fanatic, I could tell from the squeaking and rattling that he was still in beginner mode. But we got on really well and I integrated him into my circle of friends, which still consisted of the old Dithmarsch people, some of whom were now living and studying in Kiel.

I had found a like-minded person in Aron. He shared my interest in philosophical topics, but also enjoyed partying from time to time. We spent many evenings and days playing Pro Evolution Soccer on the Playstation. On the rare occasions when I was able to beat him I celebrated it extensively. We had a really good time together in the summer of 2002 during the World Cup, which took place in Korea and Japan. We both had a lot of time on our hands and watched almost all the interesting matches together. We either watched the games in our shared flat, where we were often joined by other friends in the evenings, or at public viewings in a pub. Aron knew a lot about soccer, and the fact that Germany surprisingly made it to the final gave the whole thing a special spice.

The next time I went on a meditation retreat in Bavaria, Aron came with me. I have shared this passion with him ever since. Even though he wasn't as fanatical about practicing as I was and didn't necessarily want to go on a retreat every year, he practiced very regularly and I had the impression that it was good for him and his development.

Approximately a half a year after the first intensive meditation course in Bavaria, my overall condition had already improved noticeably. Together with my doctor, I dared to reduce my high amitriptyline medication, which I had been taking continuously for over two years at this point. I was able to reduce the dose further over the next few months. At a follow-up visit, the doctor then suggested that I reduce the amitriptyline even further and also take a low dose of citalopram. Citalopram is another antidepressant that should have less of an effect on my pain level but increase my drive. The pain level slowly but steadily decreased and my overall condition continued to improve. The leaden tiredness that used to haunt me well into the afternoon and this permanent twilight state, which clouded everything, also gradually subsided.

This also made studying much easier for me. Especially when I had exam periods and had to study for days on end, I meditated extensively before the study sessions. Then I was able to concentrate better, had a better grasp of things and remembered the material more reliably.

Beeping noises

One morning, I was surprised by a new phenomenon. As always, it took a while before I could bring myself to get up. I pressed the snooze button once or twice. On the third ring, I sat up in bed and tried to assess my condition. It wasn't so good at the moment. In the middle of the break after the summer semester, I had caught a nasty cold with a cold, sinusitis and a headache. It was all mucous and even worse than yesterday, I realized. My nose was stuffy, my head hurt, and what was that? Something was beeping. A bright, constant beeping in my left ear. It sounded like after a metal concert, except that I hadn't been to a concert or a student party in the last few days. It was beeping quite loudly, but I tried to ignore it for the time being. I went to the bathroom and then to the kitchen to make myself a coffee.

"Good morning Aron, you're already awake. Did you sleep well?" I grumbled when I saw my flatmate.

"Yes, quite well. And you, are you feeling better today?"

I had trouble understanding him. It sounded like he was speaking through absorbent cotton.

"Uh, I can't hear you very well, maybe I have something in my ear or something. Hang on, I'll turn to the other side, maybe I can hear better with the other ear. Say something again."

"Yes, what can I say, can you hear me?"

"Hm. Yes, I can hear much better on the side. That's strange."

It was beeping in my left ear, and I could only hear at about half the volume there. That was already a bit scary. Was it just the loud beeping, or was my hearing also weaker? I decided to take it to the emergency room instead, as it was Sunday and the normal doctors' surgeries were closed.

At the university hospital, they diagnosed a sudden hearing loss with tinnitus in my left ear. I was hospitalized for a week and received infusions every day. Apart from my severe cold, I didn't feel ill at all. It was strange to be in hospital as a virtually healthy person. The attending doctor asked me if I had been to a concert or if I was under a lot of stress. I denied both. My neck pain and headaches were still bad, but they were clearly on the mend. I liked my subjects in my main course and felt comfortable in the shared flat. I was also on semester break and meditated a lot. In contrast to my previous life, my stress level was currently rather low, although the pain was of course still a major stress factor. I asked if the cold could have caused the sudden hearing loss. The doctor replied that this was rather atypical. So once again a mystery without a recognizable cause. I found this unsatisfactory, so I did some more research myself.

The following possible causes were also mentioned on the Internet: "Inflammation of the ear, viral and bacterial infections or functional disorders of the cervical spine". Both of the latter were true, and that sounded more like a plausible explanation to me.

Especially at the beginning, it beeped so loudly that it really bothered me and I was afraid that it would stay that way permanently. This constant beeping could drive you mad!

Fortunately, labeling helped me enormously here. I labeled

"hearing, hearing,hearing" and sometimes "worrying, worrying, worrying" and realized that I could then accept the beeping much better without losing myself in aversion, worry and anxiety about it.

After a few weeks, I regained my full hearing and the tinnitus slowly subsided. However, it took months before it was so weak that I only noticed it very rarely - until I almost forgot it existed.

The enthusiasm is growing

For my studies, I read thick tomes of specialist literature on business management topics and information technologies.

In the course of my main studies, I became more and more enthusiastic about software. I found the complexity and power of programming languages fascinating. In my software engineering seminar, I learned that software was usually developed in a complex, iterative process. First, you had to clarify the technical requirements with the client and design a data model based on this. This was then refined in several rounds based on workshops and close collaboration between all those involved until it met all requirements. It was not only important to correctly understand and interpret the technical requirements, but also to develop a suitable data model. In addition, the desired functions had to be considered in relation to the complexity and effort involved and the technical restrictions and capabilities of the project team. It was therefore an extremely dynamic and complex process that also required a good deal of negotiating skill. I found this mixture very interesting. I found the role of a system analyst the most exciting. He had to design the software system, take responsibility for its architecture, but also weigh up the requirements of the specialist department against the technical possibilities. He therefore had to understand the programmers and the programming language, but also the technical requirements. So software analyst became my dream job.

I could live out my technical fascination, but also have a certain amount of human interaction due to the role. I liked this relationship. However, my new career aspirations also meant that I had to acquire a huge amount of technical knowledge to get that far. I also wasn't sure if I could muster the linguistic ability and confidence to interact with multiple parties on such a complex level.

In our Software Engineering course, we had to present the system design that we had developed in our groups over several weeks in a presentation in front of the other students and stakeholders from a real business company. I was very excited during this presentation and my heart was pounding while I was presenting. I could barely read what was on my slides - that was all I could manage. My head was foggy with excitement and anxiety. I was miles away from a free, relaxed presentation. Although I had significantly more knowledge than the other members of my project team, I delivered the worst performance. I hoped that this would improve over time. At first, I left it at the idea that working as a software analyst was still a distant dream.

Vipassana studies

Over time, I bought various books on meditation, Buddhism and especially Vipassana meditation, most of which I bought cheaply on eBay. I spent a lot of time devouring these books and became a real bookworm. I wanted to find out more about what I had experienced, what I was still experiencing and where it would take me.

By now I had a real little collection of books in my cupboard. Many people joke about the state of enlightenment, but hardly anyone really knows what it actually means. I was intrigued when I found a book that explained enlightenment in Theravada Buddhism in more detail. Since I now considered myself a Buddhist, I definitely wanted to know exactly.

Of course, I was also interested in how much more meditation I would have to do before I was enlightened myself, and what that would feel like.

Buddhism mentions six realms of existence. There are two realms of the gods, the devas and the titans. These are followed by the realm of humans and the realm of animals. Then there is the realm of hunger spirits. These are spirits who have to suffer constant hunger and thirst due to their karma. Finally, there is the realm of hell with its infernal beings. The beings in hell suffer unimaginable torment until the negative karma that led them there is removed.

According to philosophy, there are four levels of enlightenment. Someone who has reached the first level of enlightenment, i.e. the first level of holiness, is called a Sothapanna. The event that makes him a Sothapanna is called stream-entry. A sothapanna has successfully passed through all the vipassana yanas, or stages of insight, and has a very deep insight and profound understanding of the three characteristics of existence: impermanence, suffering and non-self. He no longer has any doubts about Buddha, Dhamma and Sangha. This means that he firmly believes in the path of the Buddha, in karma and rebirth and that it is possible to break out of the cycle of existence. He also respects and values the community of the Buddha's disciples, who have kept his teachings alive for thousands of years. A Sothapanna is reborn a maximum of seven times before reaching Nibbana. Once one has reached the level of Sothapanna, one is guaranteed liberation. The only question that remains is how many more lives it will take. A Sothapanna is no longer reborn in the lower realms of existence as an animal, hunger spirit or hell being.

The second level of enlightenment, sakadagami, means once-returner. A sakadagami is reborn once again in the realm of the senses, provided he does not become an anagami in this life.

The third level of enlightenment, anagami, meant non-returner. An anagami is not reborn in a human realm of existence, but in a pure land where only anagamis live. There he finally attains full enlightenment, arahatship. An anagami has an advantage over a sakadagami in that he has not even the slightest skeptical doubt about the Buddhist teachings, that he has hardly any sensual desires and has no predispositions for any form of hostility.

The fourth level of enlightenment is that of the arahant. An arahant has attained perfect enlightenment, i.e. realized Nibbana, by following the teachings of the Buddha. An arahant is free from all mental defilements such as greed, hatred and delusion. He has escaped the cycle of existence and, when he dies, will not be reborn, neither in the human world nor in any other realm of existence.

Compared to an arahant, a Buddha is a being who possesses even greater spiritual perfections (paramitas) and has found complete enlightenment through his own efforts. He is also able to teach and spread the path to enlightenment so successfully that many beings can follow his path. Buddhism assumes that there were Buddhas before the Buddha of our age and that there will be other Buddhas in the future. When the teachings of our Buddha Siddartha Gautama have completely disappeared, the next Buddha of the future (Maitreya) will follow and set the wheel of teaching in motion again.

INTERNSHIP IN CHENNAI - INDIA INTENSIVE

A bold step

I had prepared intensively for the interview at AIESEC. AIESEC is an organization that arranges internships for students worldwide. I had spent days researching typical interview questions, preparing my answers and writing them down. Then I went through them again and again until I could almost memorize them. On the day of the interview, I meditated for four hours so that I was ready for the appointment. Meditating had significantly reduced the pain level so that the pain was only lurking in the background and I now had a reasonably clear head. This worked better on some days and worse on others, but today the long meditation session fortunately had an extremely positive effect.

Nevertheless, I was extremely nervous. The appointment was important for me and I hated job interviews. Hopefully I wouldn't have a racing heart or black out today, and hopefully there wouldn't be so many people to speak in front of.

"Hello, I'm Nina from AIESEC," said the young woman in suit trousers, blouse and jacket, who welcomed me and held out her hand.

"Hi, I'm Philip, I wanted to go for an interview for an internship abroad."

"Then you've come to the right place! You're welcome to sit down. It'll be a little while yet." She pointed to an armchair in the waiting room and sat down next to me. "Are you excited?" She probably realized straight away that I was more excited than average. I liked her and the fact that she was talking to me calmed me down a little.

"Yes, a little," I replied.

"You don't need that at all. I'm also taking part in the interview, as well as Matthias and Nico, who are conducting the interview. Both of them are also with AIESEC."

"Okay, and how does that work?" I asked.

"We'll introduce ourselves and our internship program, and then you can introduce yourself. After that, we'll ask you a few questions, and of course you can ask questions too. But we're all very relaxed, don't worry. But now I have to go back in, there's another interview going on. You can do it afterwards."

This preliminary small talk had actually helped me to keep my nervousness in check to some extent. I even managed to present my part of the presentation, which I had practically memorized, quite well and fluently.

"And why do you want to do an internship abroad?" Nico, who conducted the interview, asked me.

"I would like to work as an intermediary between management and IT specialists later on, as my mixture of business administration background and my enthusiasm for IT means that I am well equipped for this. I would like to do an internship in India if possible. On my first trip to India, I was so fascinated by the country that I would like to delve deeper into this exotic land. I would like to find out how people really live there and get to know the culture even better. And since India is very advanced in the field of information technology, I thought I could combine my two interests quite well. But if India doesn't work out, another country would also be an option. I am generally interested in other cultures."

At the end of the appointment, I was surprised by my own performance. I had done quite well and hadn't stuttered at all. It felt like a small miracle. Without the four hours of meditation, I was convinced that things would have gone very differently.

A week later, I was approved for the placement process. As the IT industry in India was highly developed, there were indeed many choices for interns. Much to my delight, I finally landed an internship in Chennai, South India.

Arrival in Chennai

At the airport in Chennai, I was met by two Indian students who were part of the local AIESEC committee. I recognized them by the sign they were holding up. "Hello, I'm Ajay and this is Bikash. Welcome to India!" said one of them, immediately extending his hand to me. "Did you have a good trip?"

"Yes, the trip was okay, just a bit jet-lagged," I replied.

"Come with me," said Ajay. "We're here by car. We're going to Bikash's for now, and from tomorrow you'll be staying with my family. We have a room available. A Japanese man is already living there."

It immediately felt good to be back in India, even though I was actually pretty exhausted from jet lag.

Ajay lived with his family in a house in the city center. In addition to Ajay, the household included his father, his mother, his sister Anisha and a domestic help who also lived there. The family originally came from Kerala and was Christian. This meant that they belonged to a minority in Chennai, as most people here were Hindus. Ajay and his relatives sang Christian songs every evening. They belonged to the middle class and were able to send their children to good schools. Eight-year-old Anisha spoke even better English than I did. I felt warmly welcomed and well looked after for quite a while.

When I came home late one evening, I almost stumbled over a curled up something on the floor. It wasn't until my eyes adjusted to the darkness, I realized that it was the pretty 18-year-old maid who was apparently sleeping on the hard stone floor in the living room. The poor girl had no bed, not even a blanket. I was shocked!

I then spoke to several work colleagues about it, who explained to me that sleeping on the floor was relatively common in India. Besides, she would probably have a much better life with her family than in the slums where the domestic helpers originally came from. Unfortunately, she couldn't speak English and I couldn't talk to her. As I found her very pretty and likeable, I made an effort to learn a few words of Malayalam and bought a textbook. But that turned out to be too difficult. In the end, I contented myself with simply smiling at her in a friendly manner.

My room-mate's name was Tadashi, he was from Tokyo and was doing a marketing internship. At home in Tokyo, he was also part of the AIESEC team. He made a nice impression on me, but it wasn't easy to have a longer conversation with him. His English wasn't particularly good, he only ever spoke when asked and then only replied in short sentences.

Internship in technical support

I worked for Slash Support. The company ran a large call center and specialized in technical support. They had several hundred employees and the office looked ultra-modern. Their customers included well-known American brands such as Cisco, SUN and VMWare.

Our team provided second-level support for Alcatel eCommunication servers. These were a combination of a telephone system and a small web server, which were mainly used in small and medium-sized companies. It was a pilot project, as the support was provided by Indian call center agents in German, English, French and Spanish language. We supported Alcatel-certified technicians if they had problems that they could not solve on their own.

I enjoyed familiarizing myself with the complex subject matter and understanding more and more of it. We always worked on the problems as a team and I got on well with my Indian colleagues. They were all very nice and I liked them. After a while, I was even allowed to work on problem cases on my own, which filled me with pride. However, I still had considerable problems with headaches and neck pain and often felt that I was at the limit of my capabilities in view of the demands.

To be on the safe side, I had my GP prescribe me tetrazepam again at home. The tablets relaxed the muscles and had an anxiety-relieving effect. I had been given them for a short time a few years ago and they had worked quite well. Unfortunately, you could become addicted to them and the more often you took them, the less effective they became. For this reason, I only took them when I really felt it was necessary, i.e. when I was in particularly severe pain and felt really bad. But the tablets did a good job of bridging the gap, as otherwise I sometimes simply wouldn't have been able to get through a ten-hour working day.

Cultural differences

I got on well with my host family, but after a while I realized that our lifestyles could hardly be more different. I had quite unusual working hours, as I worked during German business hours. I started at midday and my working day went on until 10pm. Sometimes I went out with the other interns, who came from France, Peru and Venezuela, I would have dinner and a drink with them, or I would visit them in their shared flat. Six of the AIESEC interns lived there together, and the apartment was also a social meeting place for all of us.

When I came home late after such an evening, my host family and my roommate were already asleep. I then had to ring the doorbell, the dog would start barking loudly, waking up half the neighborhood, and usually the mother would open the door for me, sleepily dressed in her nightgown. When I was out at the weekend, my Indian family always wanted to know exactly who I was meeting, what we were doing there and when I would be back home. I'm sure they only meant well, and the customs and traditions were completely different from those in Germany, but it made me feel constricted.

I also had no real privacy, as I had to share the room with Tadashi. And our different working hours made things complicated. Tadashi often wanted to turn off the light and go to sleep after I had just come home from work. But the worst thing for me was the lack of privacy, as I didn't have enough time to meditate. I realized how much I missed it and how the negative emotions overwhelmed me when I didn't practice enough. I then had great difficulty expressing myself in a chosen and appropriate way. I couldn't really have a proper conversation or interact socially.

Not having a place to retreat and meditate had become the greatest torture I could imagine.

House hunting in Chennai

After a few weeks, I therefore decided to organize a shared apartment. I asked my Mexican internship colleague Mauricio if he would be interested in looking for an apartment with me. He was also unhappy with his current accommodation.

Shortly before that, I had bought a small motorcycle, a Yamaha with 80 hp. I hoped to be more independent with it. I was also annoyed by the daily negotiations with outrageous rickshaw drivers who never tired of charging foreigners exorbitant prices. I argued with them too often. I had never ridden a real motorcycle before, but I knew how to ride a scooter.

The weekend of looking for an apartment turned out to be highly adventurous, as I used my barely existing motorcycle riding skills to carry Mauricio on the back seat and daringly navigate through the crazy traffic of the metropolis. There seemed to be very few traffic rules. The larger vehicle always had right of way, and sacred cows were regular participants in the traffic. The narrow streets were often jammed and progress was slow. I had an advantage here with my small, agile motorcycle and was able to weave my way through everywhere.

We visited several apartments and spoke to some of the landlords. Once we were asked if we ate meat and wanted to cook it in the apartment. The owners were very religious Brahmins. They ate vegetarian food themselves and did not tolerate meat being prepared in the apartment. At the end of our tour, we were somewhat disillusioned. Most of the apartments did not meet our expectations and the rents were still relatively high. As I wasn't very familiar with the neighborhoods, we had also looked at some apartments in very remote areas. At least it had been exciting!

A few weeks later, I moved into my Peruvian work colleague Hector's shared flat instead, where a room became available. I now finally had my own room and had much more time to meditate in the mornings and at weekends. That improved my emotional situation a little. As we didn't start work until 12:30, I had time for other things in the morning. Above all, I meditated in my room for an hour every morning.

Acupuncture, the second

After some time, I looked for an Indian doctor who specialized in acupuncture. I visited his practice twice a week and had acupuncture needles inserted. I had already tried acupuncture once in Germany without success. However, I was still fundamentally impressed by the concept of energy flows and their regulation through the insertion of needles. I thought that Asian practitioners might have a different approach to this topic. In addition, the sessions were so cheap that I could afford significantly more treatments here than in Germany.

Sometimes I felt a little better after the sessions, but overall there was no positive effect, so I stopped the treatment after about 20 sessions, disappointed. That was therapy attempt number ten.

I kept both my visits to the doctor and my intensive meditation sessions secret from my flatmate Hector. I was so uncomfortable with this whole topic that I didn't want to get involved in conversations about it. I still felt like it would be too hard for other people to understand and too hard for me to explain why and how I was meditating and seeing doctors so much. Maybe I was also afraid of being stigmatized again.

Motherland Yoga

Having been to the motherland of yoga before, I naturally wanted to try it out of curiosity. Maybe it would also help with the pain.

After a while, I found a yoga class nearby. It took place in the city center, which was only 15 minutes away on my motorcycle, and was led by an Indian. He taught Hatha Yoga and explained it quite well in English. However, the course started at the crack of dawn at 6.30 a.m., so I visited him sometimes more, sometimes less. The teacher was friendly, funny and reasonably professional, as far as I could tell. During the yoga class, the mosquitoes attacked me persistently every time, and I kept bringing home a few new mosquito bites.

I was usually so tired afterwards that I went straight back to sleep and was pretty much thrown off my rhythm. Although I attended yoga classes several times a week for several months, I was unable to achieve any noticeable improvement in my pain through this measure either. Another futile attempt, now number eleven.

Socializing in India

I liked the mix of Indian work colleagues, the other AIESEC interns from all over the world and my intern work colleagues from Slash Support, most of whom were from Latin America. We often went out to eat together as part of the AIESEC intern community and also went on more and more weekend trips together. There was a great sense of community in our group.

At Christmas, we celebrated together with many different nationalities in the AIESEC flat share. We organized a Christmas Secret Santa in the afternoon. Everyone brought a present, which was then raffled off. Later, our Indian colleagues from Slash Support joined us, who, as Hindus, had never really celebrated Christmas before. It was extremely interesting for them to see how it all went.

There was a communal meal and everyone brought a typical dish from their home country, resulting in a lovely buffet. Immediately after the meal, the Latinos started dancing, even though there had been no alcohol, yet!

It was a wonderful evening with a great atmosphere, lots of Indian beer and loud Latin American music. Far away from home, it was a successful substitute for the usual Christmas with the family.

Sai Baba

One weekend, I traveled from Chennai to Puttaparthi, where the ashram of the famous Guru Sai Baba was located. I reached Puttaparthi by train after a few hours.

I had already heard about Sai Baba when I had first been to India. Four years earlier, I had met a young American in Goa who had identified himself as a devotee of Sai Baba. He had told me how Sai Baba had changed his life and always carried a small casket of sacred ashes with him, which was said to have a healing effect.

In recent years, strange articles about Sai Baba have repeatedly appeared in the media. He was said to own countless Rolls Royces, have thousands of followers in India and around the world and be able to materialize objects out of thin air. There were also rumors about him abusing women. My opinion of him was divided based on the information I had, but I was curious enough and wanted to see the whole thing for myself.

There were actually thousands of devotees of Sai Baba living in Puttaparthi, and almost all of them were walking around in white robes. I got accommodation for the night and then joined the thousands of people waiting to attend the evening darshan, the meeting between master and disciples. It took an hour before Sai Baba finally appeared on stage. Unfortunately, I was standing a few hundred meters away and therefore couldn't see too well. Nevertheless, I was a little disappointed. Sai Baba looked old and had disheveled white hair. There was nothing particularly lively or magical about him, at least from this distance. On the contrary, he looked rather frail physically. I didn't find the darshan ceremony particularly exciting either. He waved to his devotees for a while and then there was some chanting.

Somewhat disillusioned by this pale experience, I traveled back to Chennai the next morning.

A new romance

At the beginning of the second half of my internship, I applied for a few days off and went on a ten-day trip with Amanda and David through South India. David was a Peruvian colleague from Slash Support who I got on well with. He liked to talk a lot, and as I generally didn't talk much but liked to laugh, we were a good match. Amanda was from Hong Kong, spoke very good English and was doing a marketing internship in Chennai. Together we traveled the backwaters of Kerala, spent a few days on the breathtaking beach of Varkala and watched the sunrise together in Kanyakumari, the southernmost tip of India, where the Atlantic and Pacific oceans meet. The three of us got on really well and enjoyed the tour. I was only able to meditate a little on the trip, which was a bit of a problem for me, but overall it was great and a very nice experience.

Amanda and I quickly clicked, and some time after the trip we became a couple. It was great to finally have a companion again. I had had my last real girlfriend when I was 19. That was five years ago! Since then, I hadn't been particularly emotionally close to anyone. On the one hand, my problems made it difficult for me to express myself and make really close contact with anyone. On the other hand, I didn't want to and couldn't really expose anyone to the immense negativity that lay dormant inside me and was poisoning me and those around me. Many people probably noticed this unconsciously and involuntarily kept their distance from me. Since I started meditating, however, I felt a bit more emotionally stable and balanced again. I felt more joy and optimism in life again and was now ready to let someone get closer to me.

I enjoyed my time with Amanda. We got on well and even went on a trip together as a couple through India. Amanda did most of the planning. As a result, we visited as many sights as possible in as short a time and took lots of photos. In three weeks, we went from Chennai to Goa, to Udaipur, to Agra to the Taj Mahal, to Delhi, to Varanasi on the holy river Ganges and finally to the mountains of the Himalayas to Darjeeling. There we admired the tea plantations, which stretched as far as the eye could see. At the end, we returned to Chennai via Kolkata with a one-day stopover. It was a crazy and exhausting tour, during which my MP3 player was stolen on the train. But it was also a beautiful and unforgettable journey. On the multi-day train journey from Varanasi to Darjeeling, we once drove right through a swarm of millions of fireflies. Their glow in the dark night was simply indescribably magical - it left us speechless.

The six months I spent in India were fascinating, amazing, surprising and, in all their chaos and incompleteness, incredibly enriching on many levels. Living there forever would certainly be difficult due to all the cultural differences, but I took a lot of inspiration from India with me. Amanda and I stayed together for a few weeks after our time in India and had a long-distance relationship. I even toyed with the idea of looking for a job in Hong Kong. But in the end I rejected that idea and that was the end of our story together.

CAREER START - A NEW PASSION

Sweet Home and TCM

In the summer of 2004, after my stay in India, I lived in a small one-bedroom apartment next door to my parents for a few months. I had already completed my thesis there and successfully passed my diploma in business administration with a focus on business informatics. Now I was looking for a job. I spent a lot of time with my parents, which was quite harmonious, and also got to know my brother, who was ten years younger than me, for the first time. He was now 15 years old, liked to play soccer, went to his first parties and I was able to do a lot more with him than before. We went to the gym together a few times, to the movies and to one or two parties, and built up a real brotherly bond.

Behind my apartment was a meadow with a biotope. Countless insects crawled and flew in through the window every time I wasn't careful. Instead of chasing them with a fly swatter or vacuum cleaner, as I would have done in the past, I now caught them with a jar and released them outside. Since the first three-week meditation course, I no longer had the heart to kill insects on purpose. It wasn't so much the fear of catching bad karma as a connection I felt to the animal that drove me to do so. I had the feeling that this was particularly connected to the metta practice that I always practiced after sitting meditation. And it felt good every time I saved a little life like that.

As I had not completed any internships in Germany and as I didn't have any other special "vitamin B", I wrote almost 100 applications and was invited to nine interviews.

At that time, my mother told me about a friend she knew from horse riding. The woman had had migraines for many years and had been cured with acupuncture by a doctor from Hamburg who practiced TCM (Traditional Chinese Medicine). That sounded good, and although my acupuncture treatment in India had been unsuccessful, I still had more faith in a real Chinese TCM doctor. At the very least, I wanted to give it a try. My pain was much better than before, but it was still making my life difficult. I had to meditate a lot to keep it at a bearable level. Every morning when I got up, I was confronted again with the pain in my neck, the pressure in my head, the irritable mood. Only after an intensive meditation session did things improve. After the next sleep, however, it was already worse again. That's why I was still open to therapies that promised relief. The TCM treatment was not covered by health insurance, but my mother said I shouldn't worry about paying for it - my parents would help me. A single treatment cost 80 euros. The practice was in Rahlstedt, a district of Hamburg in the far east of the city. It took me two and a half hours to get there by car, as I had to drive all the way through Hamburg. That was a lot of effort, but it was worth a try.

The doctor asked me lots of questions about my eating habits and did a cupping treatment and a moxa session at the first appointment. During the cupping treatment, suction cups were attached to my back and left hanging there for a while. Then a needle with a burning incense ball was fixed to a certain spot on my neck, similar to an acupuncture needle - the so-called moxa therapy. During the second session, she applied various Acupuncture needles in my neck and ears. I was also given recommendations on which foods I should eat more of in future and which I should avoid.

When I had spent countless hours in the car after eight therapy sessions and had spent a considerable amount of money, but there was absolutely no positive effect, I broke off the treatment once again in disappointment - attempt number twelve.

After this experience, my desire to become a naturopath finally died out. I had already tried too many unsuccessful therapies with alternative healing practices and found that meditating helped me a hundred times better than any other therapy.

Entry into the SAP world

In January 2005, I started my first real job as a Junior SAP Consultant at Aprimus GmbH, a medium-sized management consultancy for business software with almost 30 consultants. I had some concerns as to whether I could meet the requirements of the job, but nevertheless I was also highly excited about this new challenge. First, they sent me to Walldorf for five weeks. That's where SAP's headquarters were located, where I was supposed to complete a training course and then take an exam and receive a consultant certificate as an SAP Solution Consultant. I had to learn a lot, but although the material was challenging, I passed the exam. I then accompanied some of my new colleagues to a project in Poland every week, where we supported an SAP implementation for a mechanical engineering company. My role in the project was to assist an experienced colleague who was responsible for sub-project management in the sales department for the SAP implementation. This concerned all sales processes that were mapped in the software. First of all, I took the requirements for print-relevant documents such as invoices, order confirmations and delivery bills. This proved to be extremely challenging, as there were a lot of legal regulations in Poland, the printouts had to be issued in various languages and I had little knowledge of the subject matter. I then specified the requirements so that they could be programmed remotely by colleagues in India. I then tested the settings and processes.

When I had already been working on the project for a few months, the senior colleague for my area announced that he had resigned. He had accepted a position with less travel at another company. As there was no suitable replacement within our small company, I was forced to take over his tasks and report on the progress of the project in the sales department at the status meetings. However, as I didn't have the necessary expertise to manage the sub-project, I had to work closely with an Indian consultant who was based in the USA. Thanks to my experience in India, I was able to understand him well - unlike most of the others - even in the telephone conferences. I enjoyed working with him virtually. But the project was also quite stressful and all the new terms and complexities almost constantly overwhelmed me. I was usually exhausted by the weekend. Nevertheless, I was proud that I hadn't messed up my career start and that I was even doing a good job on the challenging project.

In mid-2006, the year after I started working, I finally stopped taking antidepressants completely. Everything had improved so much through the retreats and daily practice that I felt much more stable. I was very happy that I could now live without the medication again, which had had a major impact on my system for the last six years. It was a liberating feeling. At last I was no longer dependent on these chemicals, and all thanks to Vipassana meditation!

That same year, I also had my first longer romantic relationship again for several years. I was happy and delighted with the positive development.

Living in a shared flat with Sven

I now lived with my friend Sven in a shared flat. I had gotten to know Sven many years ago when we had sat next to each other in our geography class at school. He had gone on to study Business Administration at Kiel University, while I had been at the University of Applied Sciences. But we had met up occasionally to play computer games and sometimes to study or party. Together with other friends, we had also gone on a few small weekend trips together and always got on well.

In Hamburg, he wanted to do an internship at a management consultancy while continuing his studies at the Remote-University of Applied Sciences, which he had switched to in the meantime. We lived in a small but chic apartment very close to the famous Schulterblatt. In just a few minutes, we were in the middle of the trendy Schanzenviertel with all the cafés, restaurants and bars. There was even a beach club around the corner, which became our second living room in the summer. Despite this, the apartment was quite quiet and I was able to sleep well there.

We usually went out partying together at the weekend. Our apartment often served as the base. Friends and acquaintances would come over for the pre-party. Then we'd move on to the Goldfischglas, a well-known bar, and drink mojitos or caipirinhas. We often let ourselves drift, wandered through a few cocktail bars on the Schanze and then continued partying in a club on the Kiez. Our favorite was the China Lounge. On the first floor they played cool house music, and in the basement there was R'n'B, rap and hip-hop. They also served more Cuba Libre or vodka-Red Bull. Sometimes

we then went further up the Hamburger Berg, moving back and forth between the various bars. It wasn't until the early morning that we'd had enough, so we didn't fall into bed until three, four or five o'clock. The next day, I slept until midday and spent the day in bed or on the couch, curing my hangover.

In the summer of 2006, we had great fun with the soccer summer fairy tale. We met up with a group of people for every game and watched the World Cup matches at a public viewing somewhere on the Schanze. The weather was sunny and warm throughout the summer and we enjoyed a carefree time of soccer and partying.

Goenka course

Every year I continued to go on at least one ten-day retreat. I usually opted for the summer course at the Benedictine monastery in Bavaria with Thanat and Hildegard. In 2007, however, I wanted to try something different and took part in a Goenka Vipassana retreat.

S. N. Goenka was the most famous Vipassana meditation teacher of all. He had made Vipassana known worldwide and there were over 100 meditation centers in many countries that taught exclusively according to his method. Goenka was a businessman of Indian descent who lived in Myanmar with his wife and children and began meditating due to severe migraines. After 14 years of intensive meditation practice, his teacher Sayagyi U Ba Khin had finally authorized him as a teacher, and Goenka had brought Vipassana meditation from Myanmar back to India, the homeland of the Buddha. Many large centers had sprung up there, where people were taught in the tradition of Goenka.

Many of the typical Buddhist rituals were dispensed with during the ten-day courses using his method. I suspect it would otherwise have been difficult to attract devout Hindus.

The concept and the way Goenka taught became very popular and many centers were established around the world.

Goenka's story touched and inspired me, as it was similar to my own story. My headaches and neck pain were also a strong motivation to engage in meditation and led me down this path. I wanted to know how the Goenka method differed from the technique I was practicing and why it attracted so many people.

Together with my friend and former flatmate Aron, I signed up for a ten-day course in Triebel. Around 100 people took part, who were accommodated separately for men and women in rooms for six people. There was a very strict ban on talking. We slept seven hours a night, had breakfast, lunch and a light soup and salad in the evening.

The meditation instructions all came from CD and were tailored to the course of a ten-day retreat. We always sat together with all the participants in the large group and listened to the instructions or meditated.

For the first three days, we practiced what is known as Anapanasati: we focused on the tip of our nose and felt the air flowing in and out. Every time we drifted off, we returned our attention back to it. We did all the meditations sitting cross-legged and there was no mental labeling involved in this technique. After three days, my concentration increased greatly, my perception became more refined and the distractions decreased.

Then we switched to body sweeping. We focused our attention on the surface of the body and went through it from top to bottom and back again. We repeated this again and again. After a while, it felt more and more fluid. We were supposed to perceive and observe the sensations on the surface of the body. Regardless of whether they were pleasant or unpleasant, we were supposed to consider the awareness that all phenomena were transient and try to accept them with equanimity.

That seemed to me to be the central point of the method. I found it easier to sit for long periods of time with this method. We often sat for an hour and a half and were even allowed to bend our legs to the left or right sometimes. I suspected that because of the intense concentration, distractions were blocked out. I felt very clear and present most of the time during the retreat and was able to follow the instructions well.

In the second half of the retreat, I felt the same unpleasant tensions and the same twinge in my back between my shoulder blades that I had experienced in all previous retreats. With the new technique, I was able to observe these phenomena well, maintain a surprisingly stable equanimity most of the time and observe the sensations with composure.

Although there were clear differences in the approach, after a while the same negative energy phenomena had formed as in the earlier retreats. This suggested that both methods had a similar effect despite the different approach. After the ten days, I was grateful for this valuable experience and also thought that it was a beautiful method that was well communicated. I could imagine that many people, especially in the West, could identify with the undogmatic, practice-oriented teaching. It is possible that this is why Goenka's approach was so successful.

However, I myself felt a stronger connection to my old

method and then practiced again according to the technique in the tradition of Ajahn Tong Sirimangalo, which had been with me for several years.

On course for professional success

At the beginning of 2010, I had already been working for the same medium-sized management consultancy as an SAP consultant for five years. Since then, I had progressed from Junior Consultant to Senior Consultant. I loved it, analyzing complex business contexts, specifying requirements and then implementing them in software solutions. I was fascinated by the fact that something as abstract as a programming language could be turned into a tool that people actually worked with.

While working on the issues, I developed a passion, almost bordering on obsession, to solve every problem as best and as quickly as possible. I could immerse myself in it for hours and forget about the world around me until I finally had a good solution ready and was happy about it.

I also benefited significantly from meditating professionally. I was able to maintain a high level of concentration on a specific work topic for hours without digressing and quickly achieved presentable results. I noticed my own emotional vibrations and those of my colleagues and customers more intensely and earlier and was able to incorporate this knowledge into my behavior instead of reacting unconsciously in the moment in meetings and letting my emotions run wild. This reduced my stress levels, improved my working relationships and encouraged the compromises often necessary in finding solutions. It also helped me to put myself in someone else's shoes and see the world through different eyes. I often had to abstract complex issues so that I could explain them in simple terms to a project manager or user, for example, as they had less technical knowledge. I usually managed this quite well.

I had an almost omniscient mentor in my colleague Torsten, who I could always ask if I was stuck or simply needed a tip. He had extremely extensive experience with SAP and from consulting and project management to programming, he covered all the areas that an SAP consultant could do. I got on well with him and often kept him company in the smoker's kitchen. Then I'd pepper him with questions until I smelled like I'd just come out of a pub. But I didn't smoke during the day. Only in the evenings and at weekends. I thought that if I also smoked at work, I would become too addicted to nicotine.

Sometimes we also sat together with a projector and organized our own small internal workshops and worked together on the projects. I also learned programming in the style of "learning by doing" and completed many small and larger projects quite successfully. As a consultant who could also do some programming, it was relatively easy for me to work with the right programmers to design solutions.

I was quickly given a lot of personal responsibility in projects, and customers, colleagues and my boss were happy with me. I built up a good reputation in the company as a competent and reliable consultant. I earned a good salary, drove a BMW single-seater company car and was proud of my job and what I had achieved so far.

Relaxation on the lake district

One Friday in summer, I got off work at 3 p.m. and picked up my girlfriend Anna at home. Soon we were driving my BWM on the highway towards Berlin and then on to spend the weekend camping on the Mecklenburg Lake District.

Anna's son Tobi was spending the summer vacation with his grandparents. We were therefore able to spend a lot of time together at the moment and were looking forward to the weekend together.

The sky was almost cloudless and it seemed to be the perfect weather for our trip. "Look, according to the sat nav we arrive at the campsite at 7:30 pm. Hopefully we can still check in then. I didn't think the drive would take so long," I remarked on the way. "Could you maybe see if you can find the phone number for the campsite and give them a call? I sent you the link."

Anna immediately set off on a search with her cell phone. For a long time we drove along dirt tracks and country lanes, eventually through the deepest forest and finally very slowly at walking pace across the natural campsite, which was right next to a lake. They had told Anna on the phone that we had tent number nine. We could just make ourselves comfortable and pay at reception the next day. To save us the stress of setting up the tent, we had rented a small house tent that was already set up and also contained two loungers. I mentally patted myself on the back for this, because after the long journey I no longer felt like lifting a finger.

There were a few small groups barbecuing or sitting together with a few blankets on the nature campsite. Overall, however, the campsite was rather empty. We were really far away from everyday life in Hamburg and enjoyed the idyllic setting and the nature around us. We made ourselves comfortable on a blanket in front of the tent with a beer, goofed around and enjoyed the warm summer evening and our togetherness.

We woke up early the next day as the morning sun had already heated up the tent. After brushing our teeth, we walked to the nearby restaurant and enjoyed a delicious breakfast in the morning sun. We ordered omelettes with freshly baked bread, yoghurt with fruit and coffee and shared everything in conversation. We talked about God and the world in a relaxed manner.

After breakfast, we rented a two-person kayak. The equipment consisted of two paddles, a small barrel in which we could store our valuables in a waterproof container, and a map showing a section of the Mecklenburg lakes. The map suggested a circular route that we wanted to take. It took us through five different lakes and brought us back to the starting point at the end. The guys at the rental shop said that the route would take around five to six hours if you cycled at a normal average speed. At the beginning, it wobbled a few times and we rode serpentine lines, but after an hour we had settled in and made a good team. We enjoyed the peace and quiet, the nature, the water and the physical activity. We teased and bantered with each other, as we often did, and occasionally paused to look at different water birds.

That day, I enjoyed spending time with Anna even more than usual. There was a good mix of harmony and tension between us, I thought. It never got boring with her. I liked her sense of humor, she liked to laugh loudly and she had a similar emotional range to me. Phases of great euphoria could quickly alternate with phases of great tragedy. When she was in a good mood, she could make the world around her shine, and when she was in a bad mood, the end of the world was not far away. Besides, with her blue eyes and her exciting brown mane of curls, she was beautiful.

"Can you get the map out of your bag again? I want to check whether we're still on the right track," I said to Anna, who was sitting at the front of the kayak. We'd been paddling for four hours now, and at regular intervals we'd checked our route against the route marked on the map. Until now, the coastline had always matched the drawings on the map, but now I was unsure. According to the map, we should have seen the transition into another lake. The lakes in the Mecklenburg Lake District are mostly interconnected, so you can spend days on the water. We kept coming across small electric yachts that looked quite expensive.

"What's going on, Captain? Are you at the end of your navigational skills? Are we lost in the Bermuda Triangle?" Anna teased me.

"Would you rather keep navigating? You don't even know left from right!" I teased her back.

"Hm, it looks a bit different here than on the map. We may have missed a descent somewhere. But I don't know where. I think we'll continue for another half hour and see if we can get to the other lake by then."

After about half an hour, we finally arrived at a café, which was located directly on the shore of the lake and was well frequented. All day we had only seen nature, reeds and trees on the shore. It was the first sign of civilization in hours and we thought we must be close to our destination. It was already late afternoon, which fitted in well with the predicted five hours.

We both ordered a large Alster water, recovered from our exertions and studied the map. To be on the safe side, I asked the family at the next table if they knew their way around and could show me exactly where we were on the map. It turned out that we were way off our map and must have missed a departure somewhere hours ago. The only option was to turn around and ride all the way back again.

"But you'll have to hurry," said the man, looking at us a little sympathetically, "the floodgates close sometime between 6 and 7 pm, and then you won't be able to get through.

We were already feeling physically exhausted, as we had set a fast pace and our upper arms were not used to paddling for hours on end. We frantically drank our Alster water, paid the bill and made our way back. It was now 3:30 pm, and

It had taken us four and a half hours to get there. Now we had to make the way back in a good two and a half hours. That was going to be sporty!

We set a good pace, but also made sure that we didn't exhaust ourselves too quickly. We had to take short rest stops again and again. But eventually we made it through the locks just in time and handed our kayak back in at 6.30 pm. Tanned and completely exhausted, but happy about the wonderful day together and satisfied with our sporting performance, we fell into a deep sleep in our cozy tent early that evening.

I've never been as close to someone in spirit as I was to Anna. It was perfect! When I considered that a few years earlier I had been a "mental cripple" who would never have been able to hold down a job at all, let alone find a girlfriend, it seemed phenomenal. It all seemed like a miracle to me, which I was able to experience thanks to Vipassana meditation!

Stress factors

However, the last few months have been more difficult than the constant upward trend of the previous period. I had been working on a project in France for a year now and was only in Hamburg at the weekends. As I also lived in my own room in the shared flat, I only ever saw Anna on Saturdays and Sundays.

In addition, the project was extremely stressful. As another senior consultant had resigned, I had taken over his position as sub-project manager in an extremely demanding international project. At one point, I even flew to the USA alone for a week to design software adaptations for a large distribution center and train the users.

I always had to get up at 4:30 a.m. on Monday mornings, to get to the airport in time to fly to the customer. As I usually stayed up late at the weekend to make the most of my weekend, I couldn't fall asleep until one o'clock on Sunday and often only got four hours' sleep. This messed up my biorhythm so much that on Monday I was grumpy, taciturn and staggered through the day a bit like a zombie. I longed for a bed all day, but in the evenings in my hotel room I often didn't manage to fall asleep promptly despite being leadenly tired. It usually took until Thursday for my rhythm to settle down again. In the long term, this really wore me down.

In addition, I sometimes suffered from anxiety attacks in certain situations. Although they were no longer the severe panic attacks I was used to during my student days, they were still quite unpleasant. In my role as a sub-project manager, I regularly had to deliver status reports in large meetings with lots of people. I still found this difficult and it stressed me out. On bad days with a lack of sleep and concentration problems, these situations caused my heart to race slightly due to the excitement. But with a lot of preparation and specialist knowledge, I was able to hold my own even in these moments. In the end, the project manager was so impressed with my skills that he appointed me as a sub-project manager again in the follow-up project.

In the final phase of the project, I developed tendonitis, which spread to both forearms and didn't really go away for months despite various treatment measures. At night, I had to sleep on both sides of my arms with postural splints up to my elbows. The splints were impractical and also looked pretty unsexy. Even during the day, my arms hurt with every little movement. It was then that I realized how many thousands of times a day you use your hands to lift a glass of water, carry a suitcase or on the keyboard. With every movement, no matter how small, I felt a little pain. I had to take a week's sick leave a few times. Then it calmed down a bit and the pain became less. But the inflammation wouldn't go away completely, and as soon as I started working more, it flared up again. I was already afraid of becoming unable to work.

After six months, despite various therapeutic measures, there was still no improvement in sight and I feared that the condition would become chronic. As all attempts at therapy were unsuccessful, I thought I had the best chance of recovery if I didn't work at the computer for several months and, if possible, went on meditation retreats. In addition, in the fall and winter, I frequently got protracted colds with painful sinusitis, some of which I had to sit out in a hotel room. It seemed as if my whole body was rebelling against the current situation.

During this phase, arguments and conflicts with my girlfriend also increased. Her temperamental nature clashed with my temper, which mutated just as easily into a "drama queen" in stressful situations. We were excellent at playing each other up and taking things to extremes. On top of that, I had been arguing for several months with my new flatmate, who had taken over from Sven. He often paid the rent late or not in full. As I knew that he was earning quite well with both his main job and his DJ jobs, but was spending his money on partying and drugs, I had little sympathy for this. As a result, our relationship became miserable. I only went into the kitchen when he wasn't there and our verbal spats became increasingly heated. I no longer felt comfortable in my own apartment.

I also still had this serious problem with headaches. I actually had to meditate enough every day to feel well. It always felt as if negative energy was emanating from deep within me.

It slowly rose up through my neck and poisoned my system, clouding my head and causing headaches. After each meditation session, some of this leaked, bad energy was cleared away and out of my system. This state lasted for a few hours or until I went to bed. After getting up, however, the system was always relatively "contaminated" again. Something mysterious had to happen in my sleep. Somewhere deep inside me there had to be a huge source of negative energy that was leaking. I definitely needed my daily, regular meditation sessions.

It almost seemed as if I had two personalities. When I meditated sufficiently, I was a capable counselor as well as a balanced and loving friend. I was efficient, could think clearly, had a balanced mind, could articulate myself well, enjoyed life and liked to joke. However, if I wasn't able to meditate enough for a long time, my personality changed in an unpleasant way. Then I was a completely different person - one that I didn't like so much. I no longer reacted in such a balanced way and my thoughts slipped into the negative. Then I assessed situations completely differently than the day before. I was much more likely to get caught up in negative thought spirals.

In this respect, I was basically like a junkie. If I didn't meditate enough, pain, frustration, anger and self-doubt came, and balance was out of the question.

I often had to skip my meditation sessions in favor of our weekend plans, as we only had this little time together. However, this often put me in a bad mood and made me angry with Anna. I blamed her for making me miss my meditation session and felt bad about it. That was childish, of course. I knew that in principle too, but at that moment I often couldn't manage my anger well.

Then I was also angry with myself that I couldn't control my negative emotions and took them out on Anna. It was an insane cycle!

As there was not nearly enough time left in this life plan to meditate, I felt deeply dissatisfied, even though everything actually looked perfect from the outside. I wasn't quite sure where this dissatisfaction originally came from. Was it the demanding work, all the traveling, the closeness of the relationship? Was it because I no longer loved Anna enough? Or was it the headaches that still plagued me and made my life difficult and tiring? How nice it would be to be free of it! That was by far what I wanted most of all: relief from this torment that still caused me so many problems despite all my progress.

ASIA DELUXE - SABBATICAL WITH A NOSEDIVE

Escape from everyday life

The conflicts with Anna, with my flatmate, the now chronic tendonitis and my growing dissatisfaction led me to decide to end the unpleasant situation. Instead of moving in with my girlfriend, as we had actually planned, I made a radical change. I quit my job, ended the relationship and took a sabbatical.

Together with my friend Ralle, I wanted to spend a month in Australia with our childhood friend Jan. Ralle had just quit his job in the USA. Jan had already emigrated to Australia a few years ago. After that, I wanted to make a detour to Bali and meet up with my old university friend Danny.

Then, and this was my greatest wish, I would accept the invitation that my meditation teacher Thanat had extended a few months ago at a retreat in Bavaria. I was planning to spend several weeks at the monastery near Chiang Mai in northern Thailand. My teacher was the director of the international meditation center there, which was connected to a large meditation monastery. I hoped that by spending several weeks in meditation, I would be able to penetrate much deeper layers of the mind and eliminate the cause of my pain or at least alleviate it to a much greater extent.

Emotional breakdown

When I spent two weeks in Bali with my old university friend Danny and his partner after a fun month with my two friends in Australia, I had more time to myself and to reflect. Suddenly I realized that I missed my ex-girlfriend terribly and that breaking up with her had been the biggest mistake of my life. I wrote her a long email and told her that I had made a big mistake and wanted to go back to her. On the plane to Thailand, when I turned my cell phone back on, I got a strange text message from her saying something about an accident. I had a panic attack on the plane because I was so worried. At the airport in Bangkok, I bought a Thai sim card and called her.

"Are you all right? Have you had an accident? I was so

worried." "Yes, I'm fine, I haven't had an accident. Maybe that was an old text message from me? I'm teaching right now, but we can talk for a minute. How are you?"

"Did you read the email I sent you the day before yesterday?" I asked. "Anna, I've only just realized what I did and what we had together. It was the worst mistake of my life that I broke up with you! I still love you more than anything and I miss you so much! I would love to come back to you. Do you still want me, do you still see a chance?"

"Philip, yes, I read your email. But it's been four months since you broke up with me. My life has moved on, I've met someone. I have a new boyfriend and I'm even planning to move in with him in Munich in two months. I'm sorry. Do you remember how we stood in the stairwell back then and I said that there would be no going back if you left now?"

At this point, I burst into tears. My world shattered into a thousand pieces and I started sobbing out loud.

"Philip, don't be so sad. I'm really sorry, but it's too late."

"But you're the love of my life, Anna! I'll never find another one like you! I'm so stupid that I've only just realized that. I thought my dissatisfaction was to do with us, but it wasn't. It was the pain and the stress of work. They constricted me so much that I was no longer happy. It wasn't because of us. But I only understood that now."

"Philip, everything will be fine. You'll definitely find someone again. Please don't be so disappointed."

I could still feel the familiar connection between us and I missed her immensely. It was still so nice to hear her warm voice. I was afraid she would hang up, because then she would probably be gone forever.

"Do you love him, your new boyfriend?"

"Yes, I do, otherwise I wouldn't be moving to Munich. Philip, I have to get back to teaching. Don't be sad. Please.

Everything will be fine."

"Yeah, okay. Take care, Anna."

I sat miserable and alone, sobbing and crying on my backpacker backpack at the airport in Bangkok. My heart was broken, and I was responsible for it myself. How infinitely stupid of me! I had destroyed my own life and the love of my life.

Some moments in life feel like turning points. They have the potential to steer a life in a completely different direction. This was such a turning point. I felt that ending the relationship with Anna had been a decision in my life that I would struggle with for a long time to come.

Arrival in Chom Thong

I flew from Bangkok to Chiang Mai. When I arrived at the monastery in Chom Thong, I experienced possibly the worst day of my life. The son of my teacher Thanat, picked me up from the airport in Chiang Mai and we drove for an hour and a half by car. By the time we reached the monastery, it was already dark.

"Did you bring white clothes?" he asked me before I got out of the car.

"Yes, I have a pair of pants and a few tops. But I'd probably have to buy or borrow a few more things, if that's possible."

"Today is Buddha Day, everyone is chanting in the evening. I'll show you to your room. You can change quickly and then I'll take you to the chanting," he explained.

He then showed me the way to the main building of the monastery, where a ceremony was taking place. There were several hundred people in the hall, sitting on the floor and chanting Buddhist verses. An elderly monk was sitting in front of the assembly and I guessed that he must be the venerable Ajahn Tong Sirimangalo. He was the abbot of the monastery and the main teacher of our lineage. Thanat's son pointed his finger at a group of western-looking meditators and told me to sit down.

A little unsteady due to the unfamiliar surroundings and still foggy from grief and pain, I made my way through the people sitting on the ground and fought my way to the group of western meditators sitting relatively far forward near the elderly monk and participated in my first ceremony of my stay.

I was alone most of the time in the monastery. Thoughts of heartbreak kept coming up, wanting to drag me down into the depths like a dark, black vortex. Surprisingly, I managed quite well to stay in the present moment using the meditation technique and not let myself be dragged into the depths of my dark emotional world. Immediately when a thought of this kind came and I became aware of its heaviness and intensity, I labeled it "thinking, thinking, thinking" and went with my attention back to my current activity. If I didn't realize it until a little later and the thoughts had already created a feeling of sadness, I would say "sad, sad, sad" and then go back to my current activity. It worked surprisingly well and I didn't get caught up in my negative feelings for any length of time.

After initially doing a ten-day retreat in the monastery, I was allowed to sit in on the daily reportings. Most of the reportings took place in the morning. I sat with my teacher in the reporting room. Ten to twelve meditators came into the room one by one, and I listened to the teacher give new instructions or ask questions about the progress of the meditation. There was also a good dose of humor and small talk. I was interested to see that the meditators all had similar experiences and went through similar states. I could see that the process in a retreat was always the same and was able to compare the experiences of others with my own. This also helped me with my own meditation practice.

I also helped to welcome new arrivals and give them their first orientation to monastic life. Sometimes I was also allowed to give short explanations on meditation techniques. This task filled me with great joy and I really blossomed.

The tendonitis that I hadn't been able to get rid of for months was completely healed after a few weeks in the monastery.

Small pilgrimage

At the end of my stay, I went on a second ten-day retreat. When I finished it, I had the pleasure of departing with Phra Ofer - the Israeli monk with whom I did my first retreat in Frankfurt a few years ago - and another Israeli meditator on a day trip. Thanat's son was at the wheel and we drove for about three quarters of an hour until we reached a small, quiet forest monastery. There were a few kutis there, but we didn't see anyone. Perhaps the inhabitants were in the kutis, meditating all day.

We walked past the huts and came to a small lake. In the middle of it stood a small temple in the shape of a ship. Phra Ofer told us what the temple was all about. The venerable Ajahn Tong almost drowned here once in his childhood. He fell off the boat into the water and as he could not swim, he was miraculously saved from drowning. It was said that devas, angel-like beings, had helped him. He had this small water temple built in gratitude and as a memorial to this event.

The second stop after another half hour's drive was a somewhat larger monastery. We paid our respects to the abbot, as is customary in Thailand, and then walked deeper into the jungle. There we visited the cave where Ajahn

Tong had meditated in seclusion for several years a long time ago.

Our third stop was high up in the mountains. We drove for an hour on a narrow asphalt road through the jungle almost to the top of the mountain. There was a beautiful little monastery with a breathtaking view. I immediately liked the abbot of the monastery. He gave me a friendly smile and asked my age. There was a beautiful husky sitting next to the abbot. Seeing a husky alongside a monk in a remote mountain monastery in hot Thailand clashed a little with my world view. But I slowly got used to the fact that I was moving in a completely different world to the one I knew from Germany. To top it all off, the abbot lived in a ship-shaped kuti, in reference to his professional life before becoming a monk in the navy.

Phra Ofer had lived in the small mountain monastery as a monk for some time. He showed us a small cave where he had lived and meditated intensively for several months.

After five weeks in the monastery, I thanked my teacher Thanat for his hospitality and teachings and continued my journey. I discovered Laos on my own and then traveled on to Tibet. There I joined a tour group to get an impression of Mahayana Buddhism in Tibet. I was curious because I could imagine that there were some differences to Theravada Buddhism in Thailand.

Pilgrimage in Tibet

I had imagined the outward journey by train from Chengdu to Lhasa to be breathtaking and romantic. I had read in the Lonely Planet that the new train line had only been completed two years earlier and that it led over several passes that were over 5000 meters high. You would look out of the window, marvel at the snow-covered peaks of the

Himalayas and have nice conversations with your fellow travelers - I thought.

However, this romantic idea did not quite correspond to reality. In the 48 hours that the train journey lasted, I didn't talk to anyone. None of my fellow passengers from the entire carriage spoke English, and as the doors between the carriages were locked, I couldn't go looking for the other passengers in my travel group. I was also struggling with cold symptoms. With my blocked nose, I found it difficult to breathe, especially on the 5000 meter high passes. There were only two seats in our six-person compartment where you could look out of the window. Unfortunately, I could only stare at the ceiling from my bed and passed the time with radio plays and books. Sometimes I developed feelings of trepidation, but after two endlessly creeping days we finally reached Lhasa, situated at an altitude of 3700 meters.

Our small tour group gathered at the train station and we were picked up by a Tibetan guide and a jeep and driver. Our first accommodation was in a huge youth hostel. For the unbeatable overnight price of the equivalent of one euro, we got a very clean shared room with a great view of the Potala Palace. There was even free WLAN. I was quite amazed! It was mainly Asian and Chinese tourists who stayed in the youth hostel, but there were also a few Western tourists.

I experienced Lhasa as an ambivalent city. On the one hand, there was a modern, bustling part of the city, which now had many Chinese influences. On the other side was an older part of the city with old monasteries, thick walls and an original Tibetan flair. Tibetans, Chinese and Western tourists bustled around the streets and alleyways. Many Tibetans still dressed in traditional robes, especially the older ones. The garments mostly consisted of the chuba, a long coat with wide sleeves. They were accompanied by colorful undershirts, boots and hats as well as other accessories such as earrings, pendants, belts and hand jewelry.

Many operated small prayer wheels while walking, which they always carried with them, or let their malas (prayer beads) slide through their hands and murmured mantras. This everyday behavior was an impressive demonstration of how deeply Buddhism was anchored in society here.

The famous Potala Palace, where the Dalai Lama had lived before his escape from Tibet, towered over the city. Nowadays, however, it can only be visited as a museum.

Our young, dynamic guide spoke amazingly well English and was also very familiar with the various Buddhist deities: Buddhas, Bodhisattvas, demons, Daikinis and all the rest. I listened to him eagerly and tried to learn as much as I could about Tibetan Buddhism. However, I couldn't remember all the different names; there were simply too many.

On the second day, we visited the impressive Potala Palace and a few other temples in Lhasa together. I was still feeling exhausted from the infection I had caught in Laos when I had visited a cold, damp cave. The thin mountain air was also getting to me. Just a few steps up the stairs made me feel completely out of breath and I wanted to lie down first. I just hoped it wasn't the infamous altitude sickness.

On the fourth day, we left Lhasa and drove across the vast country in a jeep with our small tour group. Outside Lhasa, there were regular checkpoints where soldiers checked our passports and the special residence permits that foreigners needed to travel in Tibet. The houses were made of solid stone and all had a square, clear design. The people here almost all wore traditional Tibetan dress, and at first glance I detected few Chinese influences. The vast Tibetan landscape of the Himalayas had a calming effect. We drove through a rocky, rather barren and vast landscape with a crystal blue sky, a bright sun and snow-capped peaks on the horizon. As beautiful as it was, I missed the green trees after a while. There were hardly any of them here. Every now and then we saw greenhouses where vegetables were grown. Otherwise, it was difficult to make out what the people here did for a living - probably farming.

We visited many more temples in different cities and also saw a huge statue of Maitreya, the Buddha of the future. Finally, we stayed for one night at the Tibetan side of the world's highest mountain at Mount Everest Base Camp.

We spent a total of eight days traveling through Lhasa and other parts of central Tibet. The country was characterized by a traditional lifestyle, a beautiful but barren landscape and the omnipresent influence of Buddhism. As I had suspected, Buddhism in Tibet differed from Thai Buddhism in many ways. It started with the robes of the monks, who tended to wear dark colors, not bright orange as in Thailand. In Tibetan Buddhism, even light touching between a monk and a woman did not seem to be punished as severely as in Thailand. There, the monks always carried a cloth with them so that they never touched women directly, even when receiving food donations. In addition, the monks here did not shave their eyebrows.

The trip to Tibet impressed and inspired me. Even though I didn't understand a lot about Tibetan Buddhism, I could see and feel everywhere how strongly it shaped the culture of the Tibetans.

I am drawn back to Chom Thong

After the Tibet tour, I still had four weeks until my flight back to Germany. I had already had enough of traveling around and I felt that I was drawn back to the monastery. So I traveled back to Thailand and spent another wonderful, extremely intense few weeks meditating in the monastery.

At the beginning of my second stay at the monastery, I again took part in an opening ceremony to receive the eight precepts. Together with a small, mixed group of Thais and some Western meditators, we waited for almost two hours until we were finally let in to Ajahn Tong. During the waiting time, I sometimes meditated with my eyes closed and sometimes with them open.

Sitting on the bare marble floor became increasingly uncomfortable over time and my ankles ached. However, by using the practice of labeling, I was able to endure it to some extent.

The Thais were used to sitting on the floor from an early age. It didn't seem to be a big challenge for them to sit like this for long periods of time. There was also a Western meditator in our group, for whom it was obviously more difficult. He was constantly changing the position of his legs from left to right and rubbing his ankles. A Mae Chee, a lay sister, finally took pity on him and handed him one of the few sitting pads lying around.

On top of all the waiting, the air felt hot and stuffy and I became increasingly restless. I would have loved to get up and walk around. But that wasn't the right thing to do. Everyone else waited patiently in their seats and didn't move. I continued to meditate, "rising, falling", "uneasiness, uneasiness, uneasiness", "rising, falling" and so on. The discomfort increased to such an extent that a slight feeling of panic spread. Eventually, I felt like I couldn't get enough air: "panic, panic, panic".

When we were finally allowed into the room where Ajahn Tong was sitting with a few other monks, the ceremony and the subsequent Dhamma talk lasted another hour. We didn't return from the opening ceremony until late in the evening and I only meditated for a short while before going to sleep at 10pm.

In the following days of the retreat, my meditation was extremely pleasant and peaceful. I was able to walk and sit for an hour right from the start. I was surrounded by an inner calm, which was occasionally interrupted by extremely severe back pain. However, I was able to label it well and it did not disturb me at all.

As the end of the retreat approached, my condition became more and more balanced.

During my first meditation session in the late afternoon, I walked around the lake and was accompanied by a feeling of absolute peace. I heard the birds chirping and was particularly aware of the pauses between the individual sounds. My mind was quiet and free of thoughts. I enjoyed the sensory impressions, the brightness of the sun, the warmth on my skin and the beauty of the landscape. I was at peace with myself.

Suddenly, a huge hornet flew towards me and my heart skipped a beat and stopped. A violent, ice-cold shiver ran through my whole body and I felt the hairs on the back of my neck stand up. I automatically called out "fear, fear, fear".

The next moment, the hornet turned and flew off in a completely different direction. I burst out laughing! I found the intensity of my reaction to this little creature paradoxical. At the same moment, the fear vanished again and I felt "amused, amused, amused".

"How quickly things change," I thought.

In the very last phase of the retreat, I had violent outbursts of anger again. So violent that I clenched my fists during meditation, gritted my teeth and gasped out loud "anger, anger, anger". I got through these phases with a great deal of overcoming and perseverance. On the last day, I had a slight fever and a severe headache. When I woke up from a two-hour sleep at the end of the course, my heart was pounding. As a meditation beginner, I would have been worried about my health. But as an experienced meditator who had already completed several retreats, I knew that this was most likely a sign that the meditation had gone well and that my body and mind were undergoing a cleansing process.

After the retreat, I went to Chiang Mai for two days to take a short break before the next retreat. As the soccer World Cup was taking place at the time, I watched the games on television. In the evening, I strolled through Chiang Mai's Weekend Market. I felt peaceful and wide awake, marveled at the beauty of the world and was completely at peace with myself.

In the second retreat, I was able to sit with Jonathan and listen to him teach. Although he taught the same content as my teacher Thanat, his teaching style was very different. He explained many things in much more detail and more precisely. He explained many aspects of meditation with his western background in a lively and detailed way that I could understand very well. He also answered my questions in detail and I was extremely grateful to him for that.

Clarity and peace

The days after leaving the center were amazing. I picked up a few souvenirs and small gifts before flying on to Singapore for a stopover. I felt more free and alive than I had probably ever felt in my life, and I was filled with the feeling of having woken up from a long sleep. Everything I looked at seemed magically beautiful - whether it was the white cloud towers I gazed at from the airplane window, or simply the shopping malls in Singapore: there was an amazing beauty to everything, and I rested deep within myself, reverent and blissful. I felt strangely connected to the world and it was fulfilling to just "be". Time no longer mattered.

A man approached me on the metro in Singapore and we got talking. He was from the Maldives and was studying cyber security in Singapore. We had a nice chat and it was only when he asked me where I was going that I realized I had long since missed my destination. But that didn't bother me. It didn't matter at all.

I was in the here and now, and I would also arrive at my accommodation in the here and now. No need to stress.

I couldn't estimate how these nine weeks in the monastery would affect my future life. At any rate, I felt deeply moved at the moment and it seemed to me that a few things in my life would change. But that could also be due to my current joyful state of being. For example, I couldn't imagine drinking alcohol again. My mind felt so pure and clear and sensitive. Alcohol would wash away this delicate state, would make it dull and foggy again. But maybe the good feeling would fade again in two weeks and everything would get lost in everyday life.

Precisely because I couldn't foresee this development, I was excited about the next few weeks. I had a faint hope that my headaches had now gone for good. Although I still felt some tension in my cervical spine, a major blockage in my back had been released. In every retreat so far, I had always felt a sharp stabbing pain in the middle between my shoulder blades, which did not occur in normal everyday life. Strangely enough, it was the same place where I had had back pain for several weeks when I had been prescribed physiotherapy at the age of 13. My teacher said that this was bad karma. After the retreat before last, I noticed how the pain had changed and finally disappeared. Afterwards, I had felt strong shivers of energy running up my spine and I had gotten goose bumps on the back of my neck several times. After that, energy flooded my head and I walked around Chiang Mai for an hour in a euphoric but calm state, marveling at the beauty of the world.

In the following retreat, the stabbing pain was no longer where it had been for the last ten retreats, but was now in a different place. I interpreted this as a good sign.
In the morning, I left my hostel in the heart of Singapore, which had given me shelter for the last two days. I had slept well, even though there were eight people in the dormitory and a baby cried from time to time. As breakfast consisted of an instant coffee and two slices of toast with jam, I turned it down and ordered an oatmeal muesli and a latte at the nearby Starbucks. As I sat comfortably in my armchair sipping the coffee, I realized that I still had this altered perception. I felt awake, alive and deeply relaxed. For the first time in many years, I didn't actually need coffee in the morning to get me going. I had ordered it as a matter of routine. I calmly finished my muesli, left the coffee half full and set off for the airport.

I could hardly wait to fly home. What would it be like to return to my old life? Would it feel like a new life? Would it be completely without the old familiar pain and instead be characterized by this new form of alertness and clarity that I was currently experiencing? It was an exciting idea!

REALITY CHECK IN HAMBURG - BACK TO BUSINESS

Reintegration

After this intensive time in Asia and, above all, the almost magical spiritual time in the monastery, I tried to settle back into my everyday life in Germany. I looked for an apartment and a job in Hamburg. I got a job as an SAP in-house consultant at a large traditional Hamburg company, which looked great in theory. I hardly had to travel and was well paid by the renowned trading company. It was actually exactly what I wanted.

But I felt lonely and lost back in Hamburg. My relationship with Anna no longer existed and I still missed her terribly. I thought I would never find a woman like her again in this life. That often made me sad. My best friend Sven had also been living in the country with his wife for some time, where he worked in his father's tax office. We used to spend the weekends together, but that was also over now.

I no longer had any really close friends in Hamburg and it was still a big hurdle for me to meet new people. I didn't enjoy small talk, and of course it was difficult to get to the next level of a relationship without it. I also stopped drinking alcohol and meditated a lot. I no longer went to parties or discos every weekend like I used to, and when I did go, I had to fight against a lot of incomprehension. I had to explain at least five times a night why I didn't want to drink alcohol. As the alcohol level of the party guests increased, I felt more and more uncomfortable. I found most of the jokes and anecdotes no longer funny, but on the contrary felt that they violated my moral standards.

Had I now become a fun-abstinent philistine? My old friends and acquaintances also seemed to find it a bit strange that I no longer drank alcohol. We moved a little further apart. As I didn't go to parties or other drinking occasions as often as I used to, meetings became less frequent and a certain distance built up.

This was probably a completely natural process that takes place in the course of life when you develop different interests and move in different directions. But it was particularly painful for me at this stage of my life, as I didn't currently have a girlfriend and I also lacked close friends who shared the same interests or values.

To make matters worse, I didn't enjoy my new job at all. I had to show up for work in a suit and tie and sat in an open-plan office with 40 people. It all felt stiff and conservative. I was by far the youngest person in the whole department. I soon realized that I was reluctant to go to work. I felt out of place at this point in my life, both personally and professionally. I was uncomfortable in my own skin.

The headaches hadn't disappeared either, as I had hoped in Singapore. But at least they were no longer such a big issue. Instead, I was now overwhelmed by negative emotions. They seemed very intense. I worried a lot about the future, felt bad on the way to work, had no energy and was also afraid of meeting new people. I developed doubts about everything. All doors seemed closed to me and that paralyzed me. I received very little positive feedback in all areas of my life and didn't really know what I could change to make things better.

Once, during a visit to the hairdresser in Thailand, I mentioned that I had been meditating for many years and had just had spent several weeks in the monastery. The hairdresser almost freaked out with awe and enthusiasm. That was actually the usual reaction in Thailand: you got a lot of credit for seriously meditating and practising Dhamma. In Germany, I tended to get rather puzzled reactions, ranging from a mild smile to speechlessness and incomprehension. People had to have a certain degree of open-mindedness to find it cool. Apparently, my environment was not as cosmopolitan as I would have liked. My lifestyle also seemed to be more of a disadvantage than an advantage when it came to dating.

So I decided to hide this side of myself for the time being. I felt like a freak. This also took its toll on my self-confidence, because my meditation practice and my enthusiasm for Buddhism was actually a very important part of me that I would have liked to be proud of. But I hadn't managed to integrate the valuable experiences I'd had in the monastery in Thailand into my life in Germany in a meaningful way. On the contrary: it felt like worlds were colliding!

Just a few months ago, I had thought that everything would finally become easier. Unfortunately, that was a big mistake.

Startup in Berlin

Before the end of my probationary period, I resigned from the Hanseatic company in March 2011 and became a co-founder of an IT start-up that Ralle, my good old school friend in Berlin, had just founded with another friend. The two of them were initially financed for a year by a start-up grant and had now found business angels - investors who financed the development of an internet platform.

I rented out my apartment in Hamburg for six months

and moved into a shared flat for two in the same street as my friend Ralle in Berlin-Prenzlauer Berg. We worked in his living room, and as product manager I was responsible for front-end development in a team of up to ten people.

It was great to work together with a team of open-minded people of roughly the same age on an idea and develop it further. However, there were also a lot of hurdles. Programming the website was very challenging and complex, as it involved connecting automated asset management to a broker system. In addition, the new business model had to be cleared with Bafin, the German Federal Financial Supervisory Authority. The company had to involve expensive lawyers for this. In addition, our team was spread across Germany and we worked remotely with Skype conferences for a large part of the time.

It turned out to be more challenging for me than I thought, as I was not familiar with the web technologies used and had to learn everything from scratch. The banking and investment sector was also new to me and I first had to get to know all the processes. That often frustrated me a lot. It took energy and time to familiarize myself deeply enough to experience a similar sense of achievement as in my SAP jobs. My stress level was constantly above the limit. As a result, I couldn't really enjoy my time in Berlin, even though Berlin fascinated me with all its creative and artistic impulses.

I had also invested a not inconsiderable sum in the company, which was equivalent to all my savings. At the same time, I was only earning enough to just about make ends meet. As an SAP consultant, I could have earned a handsome salary in comparison without any risk. Despite the high investment, my shares in the company were so insignificant in comparison that I would not have become really rich from it even if it had been successful. It wasn't really all in proportion. But it was better than my previous job and at least I had made an attempt to improve my situation through my own efforts. My relationship with Ralle didn't get any easier either, as he was now my boss too. Nevertheless, I rarely hesitated to express my critical opinion when something wasn't going right in my eyes or needed to be done differently.

The positive thing about this time was working with people who ticked a bit like me and had similar values. I also found it exciting to create a brand and bring something to life. I also found the shareholder meetings and the negotiations and discussions with investors extremely exciting, thrilling and instructive.

However, when the platform had its successful go-live after one year and four months, I returned to the SAP world of work. I was now working for my old company again, where I had previously worked for five years. To return to the SAP industry, I accepted the fact that I would have to travel again. Two months later, the follow-up financing for the internet start-up fell through and the business was slowly shut down. So I had left the sinking boat just in time, even though my initial investment could no longer be saved.

Direction search

Since my last trip to Asia and the detour to Tibet, I have become even more interested in Buddhism with its various forms and meditation techniques. I also longed for community, for like-minded people.

I visited a few meditation centers and groups in Berlin. I had picked up a booklet somewhere that listed all the Buddhist groups in Berlin. There were almost 200 entries in it. I thought that was phenomenal! It probably brought together all the major schools of Buddhism in one city.

There had never been anything like it before. What would develop from this in the future?

I did an introduction to a Zen group in a dojo. The small dojo was not far from my apartment in Prenzlauer Berg in a backyard. A young woman gave me the introduction. She explained the meditation process and the correct sitting posture. I should sit upright and simply pay attention to my breathing during meditation. I should keep my eyes closed for three quarters of the time and stare into space against the wall. If my attention wandered, I should simply return it to my breath. Some of the meditators wore black cloaks. The whole process was ritualistic and rather traditional. At the beginning of the session, one of the meditators struck a gong and we meditated for 45 minutes, looking at the wall and focusing on the breath. When the gong struck again, we walked in a circle for 15 minutes in a row and practiced walking meditation. Then we sat for another 20 minutes. After the meditation, I felt clear and fresh, but it hadn't really worked for me.

I also attended a lecture at a Theravada Buddhist meditation center. The center was located in an old kindergarten, surrounded by tall prefabricated buildings and not far from my shared flat. A man with orange clothes and shorn hair gave a talk on various Buddhist topics. He talked about his everyday life as a gynecologist, but he also seemed to be some kind of monk. In any case, the room was packed full of very different people. I found the lecture reasonably interesting and took part in an introduction to meditation in the same place the following week, which, however, did not bring much news.

Together with a friend who was originally from Sri Lanka, I visited a Buddhist center in the north of Berlin for the Vesakh festival. Eight monks from Sri Lanka were visiting for the Vesakh festival and many people of Sri Lankan descent gathered there. We took part in a ceremony and afterwards there was a huge buffet. It was loud, chaotic, full of children and full of life. I liked that! Finally, I also visited a Diamond Way Buddhist center on an open day and took part in a meditation introduction. The meditation was very different to what I was used to. We were asked to visualize something. We were supposed to imagine the 16th Karmapa in our mind's eye, visualize him as accurately as possible and identify with his bodhisattva qualities. While the Dalai Lama was the head of the Gelugpa lineage, the Karmapa was the head of the Karma Kagyu lineage, one of the four main lineages in Tibetan Buddhism. Just like the Dalai Lama, the Karmapa was regarded as a reincarnated lama who was repeatedly reborn and then re-enthroned.

As an alternative to the Karmapa, you could also imagine a Buddha from which red, blue and yellow light shone towards you. As I couldn't do much with the Karmapa and found the variant with the Buddha easier, I tried that. However, I found it difficult to visualize anything at all, and at first no image came into being before my inner eye. After a long period of time, I finally saw a Buddha floating in the room in front of me. He was smoking a cigarette with relish and gave me a friendly wink. I was a little taken aback and also found it kind of funny. I had just had a little relapse a few weeks ago and was smoking cigarettes again after having hardly smoked at all for a few years.

Study of Buddhism

My flying visits to the various Buddhist movements were all interesting. But I hadn't yet found the right thing for me to join. Back in Hamburg, I continued my search. Together with a friend, I attended the Bhavana meditation evening at the Hamburg Buddhist Society and a meditation evening at the Hamburg Diamond Way Center.

Another time I took part in a Meetup group. A young woman who inspired me a lot had started a group online and was leading a chakra meditation group. She had learned this special technique, which originally came from India, during her studies in Australia. The way she taught everything was very modern, undogmatic and uncomplicated. I liked that, even though the meditation technique didn't really suit me.

Then I found out on the Internet that the Tibetan Center offered a course in Buddhism. The course was called "Systematic Study of Buddhism". The course content sounded extremely interesting and well-founded. In addition, the Tibetan Center was under the patronage of the Dalai Lama and enjoyed an excellent reputation. It was a weekend course with a few block seminars, which cost 80 euros a month. After a three-year foundation course, you could also complete a four-year advanced course if you wanted to.

I started the three-year foundation course in the fall. You could attend the lectures on Saturdays at the Tibetan Center or watch the livestream online, which was used by many distance learning students from all over Germany and beyond. If you didn't have time, you could watch the recorded livestream online later or download the audio file. In preparation for the events, you should usually read a few chapters in the accompanying script.

I usually took part in the events directly in Hamburg-Berne, as my new girlfriend lived only 500 meters away from the center. I had already taken part in the Lamrim course as preparation. Lamrim is a form of teaching and practice of Tibetan Buddhism with a 1000-year-old tradition, which provides instructions for the gradual perfection of the path to enlightenment. I was amazed at the high level of the lecturers. Some had lived as Tibetan monks for several years, even spoke Tibetan and had returned the monk's vows after a few years in robes. They all had an enormous wealth of knowledge and were able to express themselves well.

The first year of the course dealt with the basic Buddhist principles, such as the four noble truths, the noble eightfold path and the three characteristics of existence: impermanence, suffering and non-self. I liked the fact that although the lecturers identified personally with Mahayana Buddhism, they explained the views and doctrines of the various traditions on an equal footing during the lessons. They differentiated between Theravada and Mahayana as well as between the various Mahayana schools, which also held different philosophical views. While I had great respect for the teachers, I couldn't really connect with the other students. Many of them were older than me, and most of them were experiencing their first more intensive contacts with Buddhism. The approach of the course was also more theoretical, which only suited my nature to a limited extent. In the group discussions, I realized that I found it difficult to discuss many topics. Due to my many years of intensive meditation experience, I often knew what was meant on the basis of direct experience. The others tended to exchange speculations and opinions and approached the topic from a more intellectual angle.

Sometimes I felt like I was in a group that had never eaten a banana and was now discussing what a banana tastes like. I was the only member of the group who had eaten a lot of bananas. That's why I didn't find the discussion particularly exciting and thought the whole time: "Then why don't you bite into a banana yourself, then we can save ourselves all this talk!"

Consultant life

Once again, I wasn't particularly lucky at my old, new company. I was assigned to two projects one after the other, which put an enormous strain on my technical skills. In one longer project, I worked primarily on purchasing and procurement processes, although my training had actually made me a specialist in sales processes. Again, I traveled every week and often worked in my hotel room until midnight so that I could meet the requirements and have a sense of achievement. Because without a regular sense of achievement, I didn't enjoy my work. For me, it was downright agony when I had to go into a meeting with a lack of specialist knowledge because I couldn't simply talk away the gaps in my knowledge. There were some colleagues who were quite good at this. I envied them for it, because they had a much less stressful life and had to prepare much less than I did.

My professional life in particular repeatedly confronted me with my tendency to always want to please others. I didn't like conflicts because they stressed me out. If I did venture into a conflict, it was easy for a small flash in the pan to turn into a wildfire. Once my fire had been ignited, there was no turning back and hardly any consideration

for losses. Then I would fire my opinion unerringly and exaggeratedly with enormous, uncontrolled anger in the direction of my adversary. Whether it was a customer, a superior, a colleague or a friend didn't matter at all. These situations had to be avoided at all costs, because they left scorched earth in their wake. So I usually swallowed my anger, buckled down and did what the other person wanted, even if I didn't think it was fair.

Half of my life now took place in the hotel. I felt constantly stressed and often frustrated again because I felt overwhelmed in this constellation. I made several complaints to my line manager, but as the company wasn't very big, there were no good project alternatives. At the weekends, I was so exhausted that I would hide away in my apartment, just rest on the sofa and meditate a lot so that I would be ready to go again the next week. You couldn't call it much more than just vegetating. My life felt empty and mechanical. I was just trying to function. I had lost the deeper meaning. After a year and four months, I was so dissatisfied with my situation that I resigned once again.

Having previously gambled away all my savings on the start-up, I had now accumulated some money again. I decided to go to a monastery in Thailand for six months to take a serious step towards becoming a meditation teacher. The thought of this made me extremely happy. At the same time, I felt a little queasy when I thought about what would come afterwards, but that was still a long way off.

THE BEGINNINGS AS A TEACHER - A DEMANDING VOCATION

Retreat in Khorat

We took a minivan with a group of ten people from Bangkok to Khorat, where the retreat was to take place. The majority of our group came from Germany. I knew some of them at least by sight, from one or two retreats in Germany or from my time at the monastery in Chom Thong.

A senior Thai monk made the retreat center in Khorat available to the students of Ajahn Tong Sirmangalo for a course. It was located a little higher up in the mountains and was normally used by monks. It consisted of spacious, astonishingly new kutis. Many people were already there and it seemed as if the retreat was well attended.

Samaneri Silavaddhani, a German nun candidate, had taken over a large part of the organizational work and also showed us our kutis. Samaneri was the title of a novice. She had been given a Buddhist Pali name by her teacher at her ordination. Like everyone else, I had my own small, comfortable kuti. I felt at home straight away. This would be my home for the next ten days.

The next day, we gathered in the large meditation hall.

My teacher Thanat called me and a few others to join him. As it turned out, the others were also experienced meditators who, like me, had already sat in the reporting room and assisted at retreats: Hannah from England, Alex and Miriam from Canada, Robert from Germany and I had by now earned the status of assistants. I had already worked with Robert once together at a retreat at the Benedictine monastery in Scheyern with Thanat. I was delighted to see him again.

Thanat told us: "We have just returned from the annual three-week pilgrimage to India. It was a very nice trip, but the hygienic conditions in India are sometimes difficult. My wife has contracted an infection and is therefore unfortunately unable to teach. As we have many meditators here, but not so many teachers, we have decided that each assistant teacher will have one or two students for whom they are responsible."

I had two German students, Chris and Fabio. Both were a few years younger than me and were taking part in a meditation course for the first time. The prospect of teaching came unexpectedly and filled me with great joy, excitement and pride. I felt it was a great honor. As I was only teaching two students, the workload was manageable and I was still able to complete my own retreat.

It started with a big opening ceremony in the meditation hall. After the first day of meditation, I went through the three parts of the exercise again with my first two students: mindful bowing, walking meditation and sitting meditation. I also explained to them in detail the four foundations of mindfulness and the eight Buddhist precepts.

For doing this alone for the first time, I felt surprisingly comfortable in the role of teacher. I felt pleasantly confident myself and was excited about this opportunity to pass on my knowledge to two such inquisitive students. Over the next few days, we did reporting once a day, where

I asked questions about their meditation progress, answered questions and gave new tasks and explanations. I felt I was doing a good job and my students were enthusiastic and eager to learn. Teaching was also easy for me. On the fifth day, however, Fabio was plagued by persistent back pain and doubts arose.

I tried to explain to him as best I could that this was part of the process, that it was nothing abnormal and that pain was a good teacher when meditating. But his doubts eventually became so great that he dropped out of the course on the same day.

As mentioned, during a Vipassana retreat you go through so-called insight stages, also known as yanas. For a teacher, this is a kind of timetable from which you know which phase of a retreat the student is currently in. There are certain signs that can be used to recognize which yana a meditator is in. Among other things, the yanas are accompanied by certain emotional patterns. For example, there is a challenging stage in which the meditator is confronted with frustration and all kinds of doubts. This is also known as the "rolling mat" stage, as the meditator would like to roll up their meditation mat and leave. At this stage, meditators occasionally drop out of the course. I also found myself in this stage the next day. And now my other student Chris was also plagued by strong doubts as to whether the course and meditating still made sense for him.

As an inexperienced teacher in my own state of doubt, I didn't exude much self-confidence, so I probably didn't have much power of persuasion to get him to stay. So my second pupil also left. Just a few days ago, I was bursting with pride and euphoria at being allowed to teach. Now my ego had become very meek and my own self-doubt had grown enormously. I was sitting sadly on the steps outside the meditation hall when a young woman asked me: "Are you one of the teachers here?

I hesitated, after all, I hadn't had any pupils for an hour. So I wasn't really a real teacher any more, was I?

"Yes, why?" I replied briefly.

"I want to drop out of the course and my teacher is just not there."

That was a bit too much for me; in my condition, I couldn't take care of another doubter like that. Fortunately, I saw Phra Ofer coming around the corner at that moment.

"Please talk to him about it," I said.

I tried to take a positive view of my situation and encouraged myself. After all, it was also good that so many self-doubts came up for me in the retreat and that I would have the opportunity to let them go here, better than if they continued to accompany me in my everyday life.

At the end of the ten-day retreat, however, I felt refreshed and rejuvenated and had left my doubts behind. I then traveled with about 20 others to Chom Thong to my teacher's home monastery and spent another two weeks there, during which I again helped with the meditators in the temple and was allowed to sit in on the reporting. These five weeks in Thailand rekindled my enthusiasm for meditation, and the flame burned even higher than before.

TRAINING IN THE MONASTERY - THE POWER OF THE PRESENT MOMENT

A second home

At the beginning of my planned six-month stay in Chom Thong, I first went on another ten-day retreat. I was pleased that I already had some old friends at the temple: Manfred from southern Germany, the German nun candidate Samaneri Sila and Hannah and David from England, who I already knew from previous stays or visits. I was given a small room with my own bathroom in a small house that consisted of three rooms and a kitchen. Eyal, a 12-year-old Samaneri from Israel, lived in the next room. He had been living in the monastery with his mother Michal for a long time. Fate had brought them here, as Eyal had already fallen seriously ill twice in his young life.

We formed a small community of people who wanted to stay in the monastery for a longer period of time to meditate, assist and learn how to teach retreats. Michael from Germany and Tzanko from Bulgaria also lived in the monastery for several months. In the beginning, we sat with our teacher Thanat in the reporting room and listened to him teach. Then we were given individual students of our own, whom we taught in his presence.

After a few weeks, I was allowed to teach students on my own, which I again found to be a great honor. I developed enormous enthusiasm as I was finally able to live out my knowledge, my experience and my passion.

My daily routine was to get up shortly before five o'clock and meditate for an hour. Sometimes I went to the lake with my neighbor Michal to meditate in the fresh morning air. Then I would make myself muesli and coffee in our small kitchen and had a mindful breakfast alone in my room.

I then prepared myself for the lesson. I looked at which phase of the process each individual student was currently in and prepared my questions and teaching units. This preparation helped me to conduct the lessons fluently and confidently without getting stuck too often. I had realized that it was important for the students to see me as competent and confident in order to develop trust in their teacher. In a meditation retreat, it could happen that you went through emotionally difficult situations in which you questioned very strongly why you were doing this to yourself at all. If you then had a teacher who radiated confidence and competence, it made a big difference. If they were able to credibly convey that the doubts were part of the process and that it was worth the effort, trust in the teacher was an enormous support in this phase - especially if you were taking part in a meditation retreat for the first time.

In this respect, teaching was not so different from SAP consulting. Here, too, you had to take the customer by the hand when introducing complex new processes and mitigate their ignorance and uncertainty by radiating competence and confidence in what you were saying.

I had an average of three to five students, most of whom were doing a real retreat for the first time. I was often assigned the German and Russian students, and I admired the Russians very much for their determination. Not once did I hear a complaint from a Russian meditator that it was too tedious or too difficult. They obviously had the mentality to go through with what they had started without grumbling.

The German meditators, on the other hand, began to doubt more often and more strongly and to question whether it all made sense. This happened every time things got a little more difficult and became more challenging. However, if I was able to provide them with good arguments, they usually continued to practice with motivation despite the challenges.

A reporting session could last between five minutes and 45 minutes, depending on what the meditator needed to talk about. I usually spent the morning teaching in the reporting room with Tzanko and Michael. At lunchtime, we went to the dining room and ate our meals in mindful silence.

We usually met up with the other assistants in the coffee garden afterwards to chat. The coffee garden was a green oasis of well-being in the middle of the temple grounds. Surrounded by trees, you could sit in the shade and get a really good cappuccino. I got on best with David, an Englishman my age who had emigrated to Australia. He had been living in the temple for several months and was also an assistant and prospective teacher. With his British accent, he always talked very animatedly about his own meditation experiences and anything else he had to report, and we had a lot of fun together.

In the afternoons, I often looked after new arrivals. I welcomed them, gave introductions to the mediation technique and the temple rules or accompanied new students to the evening opening ceremonies that marked the beginning of a retreat. I also had enough time to spend several hours a day practicing and studying. I studied the Vipassana yanas and their distinguishing features intensively. As a teacher, you had to be able to recognize which stage a student was currently at in order to be able to guide the process in a meaningful way and steer them in the right direction.

I also read many books on meditation and Buddhism and continued my studies, which I had started at the Tibetan Center in Hamburg. As the bandwidth of my internet did not allow me to participate in the live streams, I downloaded the audio files for the lectures and listened to them. Studying Buddhist philosophy helped me in my teaching. I developed a deeper understanding of Buddhist concepts and was able to draw on this knowledge in my lessons. It enabled me to respond flexibly and calmly to questions. I took great pleasure in being able to pass on my knowledge and it often fell on such fertile ground. Sometimes students came to us who had already practiced in another Buddhist tradition. Thanks to the study, I was able to better understand the philosophy behind it, what the differences were to our Theravada tradition and what meditation techniques they had practiced there. This enabled me to develop an understanding of their needs, which benefited me when teaching.

Tasks as a junior teacher

In the evening, we brought warm soy milk to the meditators who were in the last phase of the course so that they could devote themselves to meditation without distractions. We alternated between the assistants for each task in turn. As there were currently quite a few assistants in the monastery, it was a relaxed job. Sometimes we did the tasks together if we felt like it.

There were around 25 rooms for meditators at the international meditation center, and managing the bookings for these rooms was quite a task. There were frequent changes and men and women always had to be accommodated separately. The planning was done with a large paper plan, which often had to be completely updated due to changes. The interested parties usually registered by email, and one of the assistants was always responsible for receiving inquiries, answering emails and carrying out room planning.

A Mexican meditation teacher who had been living and teaching in the monastery for several years asked me if I could create software for this. I actually found some free open source software for room management on the Internet that looked quite useful. Together with Manfred, we installed and configured the software for the 25 rooms in the monastery. This allowed us to carry the room planning with us on a notebook and make changes flexibly in the software without having to create everything from scratch. It was also possible to automatically generate a list with the arrival dates of the meditators and send it by email. We assistants could therefore check our emails on our cell phones and see whether one or more new meditators would be arriving on the respective date and in which room we should place them.

When you were on retreat, you were not allowed to use a cell phone. But as long as we were not in retreat, we could use our cell phones and computers in the monastery. The cell phones helped us to organize our work in the temple. I had bought a SIM card in a small cell phone store outside the monastery. The mobile network in Thailand was so good that you could surf the internet at top speed with your cell phone. I was able to use apps like Skype or Viber to make phone calls to Germany via the data line. I was also able to use my phone as a hotspot for my computer to work or surf the internet. As far as mobile networks were concerned, Thailand was way ahead of Germany.

During my time in Chom Thong, I also took on a few small projects. Once I translated Buddhist texts from English into German for a monk for an event. Another time, we provided all the furniture in the meditators' accommodation with a label which room they belonged to so that the inventory was not lost. We also took care of the teaching materials, made copies or created new documents.

I got on very well with my Israeli neighbors and was happy to have someone to talk to from time to time. Eyal usually had lessons in the morning and was also learning Thai. His mother was often busy in the kitchen making food as she prepared many of the ingredients herself. Sometimes they invited me over for dinner and it always tasted delicious.

Once a week we undertook small activities with the teachers and assistants. We organized welcome or farewell dinners for someone who had spent a long time at the monastery, or went on tours with our teacher Thanat to Chiang Mai, an hour and a half away. We often collected meditators at the airport and combined this with a visit to a restaurant or to run errands - such as buying cheese and bread, which were difficult to get in Chom Thong. Our teacher often returned from shopping and brought us assistants bread and cheese. These were relatively expensive in Thailand, but it made him happy when he could do us a favor.

My duties also included taking newcomers to the opening ceremony so that they could take refuge in the Buddha, Dhamma and Sangha and receive the eight Buddhist precepts. Particular care had to be taken with first-time meditators to ensure that they did not go too far against Thai and Buddhist customs and traditions. For example, it was immoral to stretch out your feet towards Buddha or a monk. When a monk spoke, it was proper to hold your hands in front of your chest in a prayer position to pay homage to him. During certain parts of the ceremony, it was customary to sit on one's heels, and later one could sit in the respectfull way and change to sitting sideways or cross-legged. In addition, women and men were not allowed to touch each other.

With the exception of the weekly Buddha Day, there was an opening ceremony every evening, which was attended by both Thai meditators and international meditators. The ceremony was spoken in Pali. Usually a Mae Chee accompanied the ceremony and a monk led it. In the last part, the monk gave more detailed meditation instructions. However, these were in Thai, as most of the monks spoke little English and the number of Thai meditators was significantly higher than the number of international meditators.

The opening ceremony was also regularly conducted by the venerable Ajahn Tong himself about once or twice a week. Then it could happen that you would sit for an hour in the tailor's or sideways seat and wait until Ajahn Tong returned from one of the countless other appointments he had every day. He also took the opportunity to give particularly long meditation instructions afterwards. It regularly happened that such an opening ceremony stretched over two and a half hours, during which most of the time we sat on the floor and waited or received instructions in Thai. I usually meditated during this time.

Sometimes I sat only a few meters away from the venerable Ajahn Tong. At other ceremonies, too, it could happen that I came quite close to him. For example, there was an evening Buddha Day chanting every week, as well as various other festive occasions where ceremonies were held. After a while, I noticed that my meditation usually felt particularly intense when I sat near the Venerable Ajahn Tong on such occasions. It seemed to me that I then reached deep states of meditation more quickly and easily.

As abbot of the monastery and a highly respected meditation teacher in Thailand, Ajahn Tong also held a high office in the Thai Buddhist order. He was one of the highest-ranking monks in the whole country, comparable to a cardinal in the Catholic Church. This gave rise to many duties. Other high-ranking monks came to visit to pay their respects, as well as countless disciples and followers. Representatives of the Thai royal family also visited him regularly.

At the age of 92, the venerable Ajahn Tong had one appointment after another from six in the morning until 10 in the evening, as far as I could tell. My teacher Thanat told me that he only rested four hours a night. When I had first seen Ajahn Tong with my own eyes, he hadn't seemed so special to me. Perhaps I had had exaggerated expectations and was secretly a little disappointed that I couldn't see anything superhuman or enlightened about him at first glance. But the longer my time in the monastery lasted, the more my respect and reverence grew for this man who had worn the robe since the age of eleven. He had dedicated his life to Vipassana meditation and the Dhamma and, with his unwavering energy, still set a shining, even flawless example in his old age.

During the months in the monastery, I felt alive, challenged, balanced and satisfied. My task fulfilled me. The mixture of the challenge of being a novice teacher, the intellectual study of meditation and Buddhism, all the meditating and the pleasant company, including occasional social activities, felt healthy all round. I managed quite well to stay in the 'present moment' with my attention. I rarely had thoughts about the future or the past. I lived in the moment, was free from worries and brooding and was at peace with myself.

Even here in the monastery, new negativity was constantly coming from the neck area of my spine, especially after sleeping. But because I meditated a lot in everyday life, almost every free minute, I constantly had strong energetic twitches that transformed the negativity into a more pleasant feeling. Most of the time, I therefore enjoyed a pleasant feeling in my body, a clear head and a good degree of serenity.

Only sometimes, if I hadn't meditated for a while, the negativity would build up and become stronger again. Then a feeling of pressure would develop in my neck, which could also spread up into my head. Then I no longer felt so clear in my head, became a little more restless and looked forward to the next meditation session, when it would dissipate again. How had I put up with it in the past when I couldn't meditate? It's a wonder I hadn't run amok back then!

Pilgrimage to India

In February, we went on a three-week pilgrimage to the four Buddhist sites in India and Nepal. These four places were revered by the Buddhists. They had been shaped by the life of the Buddha. The four places were: Lumbini in present-day Nepal, the place where he had been born; Bodhgaya in the north-east of India, the place where he found enlightenment under the Bodhi tree; Isipatana Wildlife Park in the town of Sarnath not far from Bodhgaya, the place where he had delivered the first teaching discourse and thus set the wheel of teaching in motion; Kushinagar in the north-east of the state of Uttar Pradesh, where the Buddha entered PariNibbana at the age of 80 - the stage of Nibbana that can only be reached after the death of the body.

Our pilgrimage began in Bodhgaya. Ajahn Tong, traveled together with a group of monks and many Thai lay devotees and Mae Chees. Many meditators from all over the world also joined this pilgrimage, so that we formed a group of almost 100 people in total. In Bodhgaya, experienced meditators had the opportunity to temporarily ordain as a monk, as this was considered particularly meritorious at the place of Buddha's enlightenment. I was one of many who decided to take advantage of this opportunity and temporarily ordain as a monk for a period of three weeks as part of the pilgrimage.

An hour after arriving at the Thai temple in Bodhgaya where we were staying, a Thai monk was already shaving my hair, including my eyebrows, with skillful movements. It happened so quickly that I almost felt a bit taken by surprise. It felt unusual to run my hands over my bare scalp. When I looked in the mirror, I was initially startled. Who was this person? I hardly recognized myself and didn't find myself particularly aesthetically pleasing. Without hair and eyebrows, I looked much older, I thought, and my now more prominent, slightly protruding ears didn't make it any better. But that was exactly what I had wanted in the end: to renounce the worldly!

The next morning we set off for the Mahabodhi temple with shaved heads and dressed in white. Many ordained monks who accompanied Ajahn Tong marched with us, as well as many other lay devotees and Mae Chee's dressed in white. On the 15-minute march, we encountered monks and nuns in red robes, grey robes, purple robes, brown robes and many other colors and different cuts. Each country seemed to have its own typical color. Thai monks usually wore a bright orange, but monks from the forest tradition dressed in a slightly darker orange. I found all these different traditions fascinating. In each country,

Buddhism had adapted to the respective customs and traditions, but the central meaning and philosophy was still largely identical even after a good 2500 years.

Our group gathered on a small platform under the Bodhi tree, in the immediate vicinity of the Mahabodhi temple. The sun was shining and as it was still relatively early in the morning, the temperature was still bearable. In front of us sat the venerable Ajahn Tong, who led the ceremony and started the chanting together with some monks. First, we had to take the vow of a samaneri, in which we followed ten rules.

I experienced the ceremony at this sacred place, surrounded by Buddhist pilgrims of all traditions, as a highly spiritual event that left me in deep awe of monastic life.

As part of the ceremony, the Venerable Ajahn Tong personally presented everyone with a samaneri robe, which we put on immediately after the ceremony. As with the hair-cutting, it felt a little strange to suddenly be wearing this robe. Was it still me? I had always felt slightly uneasy about uniforms. Even a suit and tie made me feel moderately uncomfortable. I also had the feeling that if I moved the wrong way, the robe would slip and possibly reveal too much. I moved very carefully and cautiously at first.

On the way back from the Mahabodhi temple to the Thai temple, we walked one after the other in a long queue as freshly baked samaneris. It was probably part of the ritual. I got the impression that everyone was staring at us, staring at me. And now there was a whole horde of beggars who were begging us directly and wanted money from us. That didn't fit into my head. I thought it was absurd! I had just renounced everything worldly. They had to know that too. I was now the one who was no longer supposed to accumulate possessions! Why did they think I had money for them? Did my robe even have a pocket in which I could deposit money?

In the afternoon, the second ordination ceremony to become a monk took place in the Thai temple. During this second ceremony, instead of the 10 Novice rules now you had to follow the 227 monastic rules and thus became a fully-fledged monk. This ceremony was also very special, beautiful and exciting. When it ended a few hours later and we left the temple one by one as ordained monks, I was still in a state of awe. The many fellow travelers had now positioned themselves in two rows at the exit, so we slowly walked through their midst. They had bundles of banknotes and other gifts in their hands and generously distributed them into our alms bowls until they were almost overflowing. The extent of the generosity surprised me.

I spent four days as a monk in Bodhgaya and then took off my monk's robes again along with the other short-term ordained monks. Three weeks had actually been planned. But as so many of our group had ordained and it was logistically difficult to look after so many ordained monks on the onward journey, our teachers advised us to take our robes off again. A monk was only allowed to eat what he was given and was not allowed to ask for it. In addition, a monk was no longer allowed to eat after 12 noon. It would have been difficult to provide food and drink when traveling.

I was very impressed by the ordination and the monastic life. I considered myself lucky that I was able to have this spiritual experience. However, I was also happy to take off the robe again after four days instead of three weeks, as the many rules inhibited me and made me insecure. I also felt somewhat controlled by others, which I didn't like. I didn't have the impression that life as a monk could be my path. There were too many rules to follow and I had never liked that. Besides, I didn't like my appearance at all without hair and eyebrows. It seemed obvious that my ego-consciousness or the I-identification were still very strong and I was absolutely not prepared to engage in this extreme form of renunciation. But I developed a lot more respect for the people who were able to do this.

During the rest of the trip, our group of around 40 people visited the place where Buddha gave his first lecture: the wildlife park near Isipatana, now known as Sarnath. We then took our coach to Kushinagar, the place of Buddha's death, and finally traveled on to Lumbini in Nepal, his birthplace. In Lumbini, we moved into a beautiful Tibetan monastery and went on an eight-day retreat there before finally returning to Thailand after a short stay in Kathmandu.

I still had a few weeks left in the temple before I was due to return to Germany. My savings were slowly coming to an end, and the longer the time away from my job lasted, the more difficult it became to get back into it. The closer the deadline approached, the more anxious and nervous I became. In the meantime, I had decided to set up my own business as a freelance SAP consultant. I was aware that this meant taking another step into the unknown and that it would also involve enormous professional challenges and effort. As soon as I thought about it, I was already out of the present moment and worries about the future were suddenly circling in my head again. That's how quickly it happened, from one state to another!

BACK TO THE WORLD - INTEGRATION INTO THE UNKNOWN

The new, old uncertainty

Already on the pilgrimage to India and during the remaining weeks in the monastery, it had become apparent that it would not be so easy to maintain the same level of equanimity and contentment in Germany and to stay in the present moment. At the best times in the monastery, I had had the impression that I had made enormous leaps up the spiritual ladder and that everyday monastic life glided along effortlessly, gently and almost timelessly. I experienced this as very pleasant and there were hardly any worries or thoughts revolving around the future. Apart from the occasional emotional upheaval, which I could see as a cleansing phase, it was the happiest, easiest and most carefree time of my life. I had hoped that everything would be much simpler and easier when I returned to everyday life after this six-month period.

But as is often the case with hopes, they are often overtaken by reality. Things didn't get any easier. On the contrary, it became more and more uncertain. Many questions haunted my mind. How was I going to realize my wishes? What compromises did I want to make? What should my life plan even look like? Did I want to lead a strictly Buddhist, meditative life, or could I also imagine leading a normal, Western life and treating meditation more as a hobby? How would I find a woman who suited this approach to life and who I also liked? Would I find her on the internet, while shopping, at work or at the next retreat where I wasn't allowed to talk? Somehow that seemed unlikely to me. Why did I still feel so longing for my ex-girlfriend? These questions often bothered me, and as I couldn't find any plausible answers to them, they drained my energy. The present moment was suddenly unattainable and the worries were huge and powerful.

I was also worried about returning to my job. I already knew from my last departure from SAP that it could be a mental and emotional challenge to return to work after a long break. In addition, I had a rather broad range of technical specializations and didn't really specialize in a particular module. As an SAP freelancer, I had to think about how I could position myself and convincingly sell a specialization on the market that I didn't currently have. I explored the options for SAP freelancers, revised my application documents, applied for project positions and wrote unsolicited applications to consulting firms. I wanted to work as a freelancer in the Hamburg area as I no longer wanted to travel. I hoped that the freelance position would give me enough flexibility to be able to go to Thailand for several months during project-free periods to continue my training as a meditation teacher.

I was also worried about money, as I was slowly running out of savings. I estimated that I would be able to get by for another three to four months after returning to my old apartment in Hamburg if I lived frugally. So I had to find a project quickly in order to have an income again. I knew that my parents would help me out at any time, but I only wanted to use them in an emergency.

I would have liked to have taken it all in my stride and let myself glide into my new future with an open mind. In principle, I could consider myself lucky to have so many open possibilities. But the fact was that my emotional world was completely out of joint.

I no longer really knew who I was and what I actually stood for. Back in Germany, I also quickly realized that my intensive meditation experiences didn't necessarily only bring me advantages and open doors. Finding a position as a freelancer in the Hamburg area was not so easy.

What's more, my friends' life aspirations suddenly seemed completely different to my own. They all thought meditation was a nice way to relax, but a deeper spiritual liberation was simply not a goal for them. That's why I found it difficult to talk to them about it. But maybe I was just overly aware of the social pressure and reacted too sensitively?

In any case, I felt misunderstood by my previous world and developed the subtle feeling that my wishes and ideas were "abnormal". I simply didn't get any positive feedback. I realized even more that Western society had completely different values and philosophies of life than, for example, Thailand as a Buddhist country. I had to realize how difficult it was to swim against the tide of general values and to realize a different approach to life away from Western category thinking. The whole system stood in my way to a certain extent, both at a professional level and in my private life. For example, when I told SAP colleagues that I had become a freelancer because I was pursuing training in Buddhist meditation, I usually had the feeling that this completely blew up their mental cosmos. There was then hardly any reaction to my statement because they simply didn't know how to comment further on such an exotic approach. So I soon avoided talking about my deeper motives.

Slowly but surely, I realized that it would cost me a lot of strength on all levels to pursue my wish and continue my training as a meditation teacher.

More and more doubts crept in as to whether it was worth it and whether I really wanted to take it on. Was it perhaps conceivable to let go of this desire and lead a normal life with work and family in the western sense? I even had the feeling that a great burden would be lifted if I could let go of this wish.

However, despite all the obstacles and difficulties, I still persisted in my desire. I had always been pretty stubborn!

Regardless of all my wishes, ideas and dreams for the future, earning money was the first thing on the agenda. My everyday life consisted of research and job applications. I spent several hours a day reading SAP books to re-familiarize myself with the terminology. I had noticed during the first telephone interviews that all the SAP terms were no longer in my active vocabulary. That's why I found it difficult to talk about past projects.

After two and a half months, I was finally successful and landed a project with a six-month contract in the Hamburg area, an hour's drive away. The job sounded quite good from a technical point of view and fitted in perfectly with my expectations. After just a few days, however, I realized that I didn't like the working environment at all and that I didn't fit in well there. The idea of spending the next few months there felt oppressive. When I then got the opportunity to start another project for Adidas in Bavaria, I moved there and accepted the fact that I would have to travel again. I liked the project at Adidas much better, both professionally and in terms of the working environment. I worked in e-commerce in an international environment with Indians, Russians and Americans and enjoyed the modern way of working with flat hierarchies. I started to find the trade-off of traveling acceptable. I flew to Nuremberg on Monday mornings and back again on Thursday evenings. On Fridays I worked from the home office. I was earning good money and was proud that I had successfully re-entered working life.

After about a year, I felt that this lifestyle was starting to wear on me again. I didn't feel at home in Hamburg, where I only lived at weekends, or in Erlangen or Nuremberg, where I lived in various shared flats during the week. My life felt torn apart. I felt that it couldn't go on like this forever. I had less and less energy, and at the weekend I often felt so exhausted that I would spend the whole weekend resting in my apartment, watching movies and meditating. I needed the weekends as a pure regeneration phase in order to be able to perform again the next week. There was hardly any time or energy left over for social activities.

My circle of friends in Hamburg had already been greatly reduced anyway. I had been working on many projects outside of Hamburg for years and only had the weekend in Hamburg available, and during my time off I had always spent longer periods in Asia. I was also unable to use my vacations to strengthen and establish social ties, as I was usually on a retreat. Many of my friends had also had children in the meantime and were following a completely different rhythm of life.

I was also unable to find a new girlfriend. I tried online dating, but the process of getting to know someone usually took many weeks as I was only available at weekends. For many reasons, it didn't really work out with a steady relationship. I felt more and more alone and isolated in my life and in my situation, but I didn't really know how I could change that. So I carried on for the time being.

From the gut

Thanks to my project, I was earning and saving a tidy sum every month, and my account had soon accumulated a tidy sum. I thought about what I could do with it. Interest rates were currently even lower than in recent years and my parents also suggested that I could buy an apartment or a house as a pension with such low interest rates.

I thought back and forth about whether I should buy a condominium in the city or a house in the countryside - and whether I even wanted to. I didn't have a family, and none were in sight at the time. Basically, I liked being independent; I had always seen a home loan as a burden. It tied you to a steady job and gave up the freedom to move to another country for love or to change career direction. It would also make it difficult to take longer breaks from your job. The argument in favor of an apartment in Hamburg was that it would certainly increase in value and I could then live in it myself at a reasonable price. The argument in favor of a house was that I could perhaps offer meditation courses there. I liked that prospect. I didn't know whether this would happen in the near future or perhaps many years down the line when I retired. But it was a nice idea to have that option.

So I decided to take a look at a house as a rough guide. I had no real intention of buying yet. The pictures on the online real estate platform showed a beautiful old villa with a large garden and mature trees. However, when I looked at the house with my friend Sven, it was clear that it was out of the question for me. The whole house would have had to be extensively renovated. That would have cost a fortune unless you worked as a handyman yourself. And I was certainly no expert craftsman.

Four weeks later, I drove from Hamburg in the direction of Itzehoe to look at another house. When I told my parents about my first house viewing, my mother was immediately on fire with the idea and asked if they could have a look around for me. My parents had actually already looked at two houses and recommended this one near Itzehoe, which I now wanted to view.

I was in an aggressive mood that day. The week had been stressful, my battery was exhausted and I felt this deep dissatisfaction with my overall situation again. I wasn't in the mood to look at a house today. What a stupid thing to have got myself into!

I finally reached the address my parents had given me and saw their car parked at the beginning of the small access road.

"You can already see the house at the end of the street," said my mother after greeting us. "We looked at the house last weekend and thought it was really beautiful!"

"Oh, I'm not really in the mood to visit a house. The

week was mega exhausting. I'm still stressed and overstimulated. But now that I'm here, I'm going to have a look at it!".

My mother replied with unwavering enthusiasm: "It's really beautiful. It's best to see it for yourself. We've already seen it. In the meantime, we'll go for a coffee nearby. Just let me know when you've finished."

I then drove on alone to the end of the road where the country house was located. My friend Sven arrived shortly after me. I had asked him to accompany me again. He had already bought a house himself and was much more familiar with the subject than I was. He also lived in the neighboring village.

A friendly elderly couple then showed us around their beautiful country house. Even the sight of the spacious building with its large garden had amazed me. The garden looked like something out of a fairy tale with its many colorful flowers, rose bushes and old trees. I liked the whole place and it radiated such peace. There were many large rooms in the house. The couple had finished everything to a high standard in country house style according to their own ideas. Everything was in immaculate condition and you could have moved straight in without having to renovate anything. When we finished the viewing after an hour and a half, my bad mood had been magicked away. I had fallen in love with this house.

Three months later, I signed the purchase contract. It was a brave, rather gut-driven decision, as I had often done before. When the project in Bavaria suddenly ended shortly after the purchase contract was signed, it suddenly felt heavy. I now had to make the monthly payments on a house and raise money. As a result, I no longer had the degree of freedom I had known before.

I also had the feeling over the last few months that my work was becoming too much for me and that I wouldn't be able to do it at this level for much longer. I was worried about whether I would be able to finance the house in the long term. The plan to turn it into a place of meditation often seemed far too big and scared me. I didn't even enjoy telling other people about the house purchase because I also had a lot of doubts about it. So at first I only told my close friends about it. There was usually little understanding as to why I was buying a house in the village on my own. I didn't enjoy having to answer the questions. It confronted me too much with my own doubts. Fortunately, the former owners lived in the house for another year and a half, so I didn't have to worry about finding a way to use it straight away.

I quickly secured a follow-up project near Hamburg. Before it began, I spent another three weeks practicing in a monastery in Thailand. The three weeks of meditation were difficult and were accompanied by a lot of frustration and anger. I was dissatisfied with my general life circumstances and this was also evident in my meditation. I felt that my practice had stagnated to some extent and was less effective than before.

DESPITE EVERYTHING THAT WAS - THE PLAGUE RETURNS

Roll backwards

In my new project, I worked for a large but medium-sized automotive and industrial supplier in the Hamburg area. I didn't have to travel and was able to use my skills to find my way around there. However, I was now working in a completely different environment to Adidas - not as international and not as modern, hip and cosmopolitan. But after a short period of adjustment, I came to terms with my new surroundings.

Unfortunately, I had been plagued by headaches and neck pain ever since I left Adidas. I blamed it on the torn lifestyle, a kind of burn-out. Unfortunately, this also triggered the familiar neck pain again, which I had almost considered to have conquered. To my absolute horror, it got worse again - so bad, in fact, that it made my work and life extremely difficult again. I remembered my time with the bad pain at the beginning of my studies, and it got almost as bad again.

My emotional and mental stability also continued to decline as the pain level increased. I was shocked because I hadn't thought it could get this bad again - after thousands of hours of meditation, after countless retreats, after overcoming so many hurdles! So had it all been for nothing? Was my illness more psychological or physical, or even a mixture of both? This new spiral of pain unsettled me deeply.

At night I was often in so much pain that I would lie awake for hours or walk up and down the apartment and only ever said "anger, anger, anger", "frustration, frustration, frustration". Sometimes I had to stop myself from screaming. Sometimes I wanted to bang my fist against the wall. Sometimes I even went out and walked through the streets of Hamburg at night, it was so painful. It seemed that the neck region was irritated by weight and friction during sleep and this triggered the pain. And the stronger the pain became, the stronger the feelings of anger and frustration became. I was able to incorporate them into my naming practice on a daily, nightly or hourly basis.

After countless visits to physiotherapists had once again failed to produce any results, I planned another time-out to meditate in Thailand. Even though I was already having doubts about the effectiveness of meditation, it still seemed to be the best approach for lack of better alternatives. After all, it had always helped in the past. I just dragged myself to work and knew that I couldn't go on like this. I wouldn't be able to last much longer with this pain anyway. If it went on like this, I would soon be unable to work. This caused me additional worries, as I now had to pay the monthly installments for the house loan. If I was unable to work for a long time, I would lose the house and would probably only be able to get out of the situation with a huge financial loss.

This time I wanted to give myself three months to meditate away the pain in Thailand and hopefully complete my training as a meditation teacher.

Love is unpredictable

However, something didn't quite fit in with this plan: I had recently got a new girlfriend and was really in love again for the third time in my life with this intensity. I was amazed at how this could actually happen in this dark phase, but it did. The first night we spent together, I was in so much pain at night that I walked around the city for two hours. A few times I had to cancel our weekend plans at short notice because I was in so much pain that I didn't feel able to make a 100-kilometer drive to the Baltic Sea or meet up with her friends. Julia was very disappointed that I had canceled the plans we had both been looking forward to at such short notice. I was also heartbroken because I loved her. When I said goodbye to Thailand, it hurt a lot to have to leave her for such a long time and we wanted to stay in touch as best we could via Skype. About halfway through my stay, she wanted to come to Thailand for two weeks and we wanted to travel together.

After several weeks in the monastery, I was actually still Skyping with Julia every day. I had bought a Thai SIM card with sufficient data volume and was amazed at the excellent video quality, which was almost piercingly sharp. Every day I looked forward to seeing Julia's face on the small cell phone screen. It was the highlight of every day and I missed her very much. She smiled at me and asked how she usually started the conversation:

"Hello, nice to see you! How are you today?"

"Not so good. I've got the same neck pain and headaches as yesterday. I'm pretty desperate. I've been meditating for weeks now and had hoped that I would feel better. But so far it's still really bad."

I could tell by the look on her face that she didn't like my answer at all. She would have preferred to hear that I was having a good time, or at least that things were looking up. It was now a similar process of hope and disappointment every day. But what was I supposed to do? Should I lie to her and pretend there was a perfect world that didn't exist? The pain was so severe that it was currently affecting my life and my state of mind completely dominated.

"What about your application, have you heard anything?" I asked to change the subject. But it wasn't really a nice topic either. Julia had applied for a job in Bonn and hadn't told me for a while. That had shocked me because it showed me that I wasn't at the forefront of her future plans. I couldn't really imagine a long-distance relationship.

"No, I still haven't heard from them. They're taking their time. Maybe it won't work out at all. Then I'll stay with you in Hamburg," she grinned.

I was looking forward to skyping every day, but it was no substitute for seeing each other in person. We hadn't been in each other's arms for weeks now, I was missing the physical closeness, and our conversations were becoming more and more problematic. The application had caused a rift and we had already had several arguments about it. Today we talked about our everyday lives for a while, but I didn't have much exciting news to report from my side. I meditated most of the time and as she had no idea what it was all about, it was difficult to share these experiences with her.

She then came to visit me and we traveled around the north of Thailand together. But in the end, the relationship broke up - probably also because she was annoyed and frustrated by my everyday pain and its accompanying symptoms. I could even understand this from her perspective, and after only six months of dating, I couldn't blame her too much.

But it hurt my self-esteem enormously. Once again, I felt inferior, downright crippled. The three months in the monastery hadn't improved the pain in my neck; on the contrary, it got even worse. Who would want to marry someone like me? Would I even have a family?

Would I be able to bring up children? How could I do that in my constant state of pain? Such thoughts plagued me greatly.

The black hole

While in my first retreats I had had a lot to do with panic states and anxiety, this pattern had gradually dissolved. The predominant, intense emotional patterns that now emerged in the retreats were anger and frustration. Lots of it. Where did it all come from? There had to be a huge reservoir of anger somewhere deep inside me - comparable to a black hole that stored an almost infinite amount of negative energy. Except that my black hole seemed to be slowly letting the negative energy out again. This happened slowly in everyday life and much faster in the retreat.

Unfortunately, there was still no end in sight and the black hole still seemed to have a few surprises in store. Sometimes the rage was so furious that I bared my teeth and clenched my fists while meditating. Instead of quietly naming it mentally, I would let out a choked "rage, rage, rage".

Then there were phases when the anger faded into the background and the frustration came to the fore. For a while, I was able to deal with it well and label it carefully. But sometimes it overwhelmed me so that I slumped down like a heap of misery.

So meditating wasn't much fun and most of the time it wasn't enlightening or peaceful at all. At least I had the feeling that a lot of negativity was coming out of me, which was good. Better than when it happened in everyday life. But the doubts as to whether the meditation was still working at all were strong.

Visit from Germany

One bright spot during my time in Thailand was when my old friend Ralle visited the monastery. He was also doing a meditation course. I was very happy about his visit, perhaps also because our relationship had not been quite as harmonious as in previous years since the joint project where he had been my boss.

As he had a family, he was only able to stay for nine days, which was not enough to complete a full course. However, he meditated diligently and got to know monastic life and also took part in the birthday celebrations in honor of the venerable Ajahn Tong's 93rd birthday.

New Vipassana teachers were also authorized as part of the celebrations. This took place as part of a large ceremony with several hundred participants. This time, several of the Western meditators who had completed several years of training were personally presented with a certificate by the venerable Ajahn Tong. And I was one of them.

It had been a long journey for me up to this point: Since I had started Vipassana meditation 13 years ago, I had meditated for at least an hour a day on average. Every year I didone or two ten-day retreats. I had also sat in on many courses in Germany and Thailand as an assistant to various teachers and had seen how the meditation process within a retreat always followed the same pattern for all meditators. Finally, I had lived in the monastery for a total of one year and taught for several months as a junior teacher and under the supervision of other senior teachers.

Trip to Vietnam with Thies

Another ray of hope was my brother's visit. He did a six-week internship at a financial institution in Vietnam that specialized in microloans for rural women. Before that, he had a week of free time to get used to Asia. As it was his first time on the continent, we first met in Bangkok and spent two days sightseeing. Then we traveled together to Ho Chi Minh City in Vietnam to spend a few more days together.

The pillow in our hotel room was too high for my neck and I was in so much pain that I put the pillow aside and used a towel as a pillow instead. I spent the whole night tossing and turning from side to side. When I woke up, I felt dizzy; my neck hurt and my head was pounding. I suspected the worst, as this was the second night in a row that had been so miserable. It was supposed to be another relaxing day of sightseeing in Ho Chi Minh City.

My brother and I first took the bus to the city center and visited the Reunification Palace, which had been the government headquarters during the Vietnam War. Despite the two ibuprofen pills I had taken, I walked around rather apathetically and didn't talk much. The palace was interesting, but with this headache it all rushed past me. After the tour, we walked most of the time, taking in the city center and trying not to get run over by the countless scooters. They were the main form of transportation here. The streets were overflowing with them, everywhere and you could constantly hear the rattling noise. Man, that was annoying! You really had to be highly concentrated, because most of them drove quite recklessly. Pedestrians didn't count for much here.

The headaches, the heat, the heavy traffic and the the hustle and bustle of the city had already worn me down. My mood was at rock bottom and every little thing was now starting to stress me out. After visiting a Chinese temple and the market halls in the afternoon, dusk was just setting in. We were just about to make our way back to the hotel when it started to rain cats and dogs. As we didn't have an umbrella with us, we took shelter under the canopy of a department store.

"What a mess!" I blurted out in a panic. "That's all we need now. How are we going to get home now?"

"Oh, no problem, we'll just wait here for a while and then it'll stop," my brother replied, halfway relaxed.

"It rains here almost every day at the same time. It must take an hour or two for it to stop! This is monsoon, it's not a short downpour like at home in Germany!"

"Now relax, let's wait a little while first."

"No, I can't wait here that long, I'm just too exhausted right now! Could you please check on your cell phone where and on which bus we can best get back to our hotel?"

"Oh man, I've been navigating us through the city all day, now it's your turn," my brother complained.

"I'm sorry, I'm not able to manage this right now! I'm completely exhausted with the world, have a crazy headache and can't think straight!"

I had become completely overstimulated. My brain could no longer absorb and process information. It was roaring with pain and overstimulation. All I wanted to do was go to the hotel, throw myself on the bed and close my eyes. Why couldn't Thies understand that?

"You know, it really wasn't a relaxed day with you today," said Thies bitingly. "You've been grumpy all day.

I can't have any real fun with you. And then I have to manage everything and you're stressing out here. It's not a vacation like this. It has to end sometime!".

"Thank you for this comment too! I'd like to see you when you're walking around in pain for days on end! Do you think you'll still be in a good mood, full of energy and up for a joke?"

I was offended that my brother had said you couldn't have fun with me. That had hit home. I knew myself that it was difficult to deal with me when I was in pain. I was always angry with myself for behaving the way I did. At best, I was simply unrelaxed, taciturn and introverted all day and at worst, I got grumpy and angry. Not really the company you want for relaxed sightseeing.

We eventually found a bus to take us back to the hotel and even stayed reasonably dry.

After I had rested a bit, I apologized to my brother: "I'm sorry, Thies. I slept so badly at night and my neck has been hurting for two days and my head has been ringing like hell all the time. I try to pull myself together as best I can, but unfortunately I'm not such good company. And sometimes my temper gets the better of me. Sorry for stressing you out about the bus!"

"I'm also sorry that you're always in so much pain. But sometimes it's not easy to deal with you. Nevertheless, I'm happy that we're going on this trip together. Tomorrow will definitely be a better day."

Apart from this conflict, we enjoyed our time together as brothers and spent a few nice days at the beach.

The three months of meditation this time, apart from from being officially authorized as a Vipassana teacher did nothing for my health. On the contrary, it had actually gotten worse. As a result, I began to have enormous doubts about meditation in general and about my path in life. I questioned my entire concept of life and pondered what I could do differently or better and what I actually wanted in life.

What was important to me? Receiving the official authorization as a Vipassana teacher from the venerable Ajahn Tong Sirimangalo himself had been a great wish of mine for a long time, which finally came true in September 2016. It was anything but easy to achieve this. It had been a long road, and only a few managed it. But now that this wish had come true, it no longer really meant much to me. My doubts as to whether I was still on the right path weighed too heavily.

All this brooding didn't lead to many insights at first. But at least I became more aware that I simply wasn't as productive as completely healthy people due to my pain problems. This may not have been so noticeable in the short term, but in the long term I was always paying for my good performance at work with my health. I realized that it would be better if I accepted this myself and took it into account in my plans even more than before.

As I now seriously doubted all my meditation efforts, I began a second great medical odyssey. I researched on the internet and read books about new treatment options for pain. To my astonishment, I still couldn't find any groundbreaking differences in therapy compared to the measures of 20 years ago, which hadn't really helped me.

The fashion industry

Back in Hamburg, I also started my new project at a fashion company. It was a completely new implementation of an SAP solution for the fashion industry, in which I specialized. In theory, I was able to put all my previous SAP knowledge to optimum use and bring it up to date, as the very latest technologies were to be used for this new implementation. The project was also located in Hamburg and I only needed ten minutes to get there. Perfect conditions! I was looking forward to this new challenge, both professionally and in terms of content. At the same time, however, I was also worried about whether I would be able to do it in my current state of health. I had therefore negotiated that I would only work four days a week so that I had time to recover on Fridays.

I was excited before the presentation, much more excited than usual in recent years. Due to the constant headaches, my overall condition was not the best. There were 20 people sitting in the meeting room, mainly men. Some were wearing suits, some casual business attire. I knew five or six of them from previous meetings over the last two weeks, but not very well. Today was about presenting the concept for the development of the IT interface to the logistics service provider. For this kick-off, a managing director of the logistics service provider gathered with a few employees and the managing director of their IT service provider, accompanied by a few IT experts and software developers. Our project manager and the technical lead of the project, both from SAP, also attended the meeting, as well as some other consultants working on the project.

My project colleague, with whom I had prepared the presentation but who was actually my customer, took on the first part. She explained the basic processes that played a role in the storage and retrieval of goods and tried to deduce which system changes would be necessary due to the introduction of SAP. She gave a fluent presentation and responded well to questions. A good start.

Then it was my turn to take a closer look at the technical part. I felt tense and it made me nervous to be the center of attention of all these foreign experts and people in charge. I was able to explain the part I had prepared in the presentation reasonably satisfactorily.

The meeting was to be followed by a workshop in which we went through the interface specification field by field and wanted to reach a rough agreement. As the project was still in its early stages, not all processes were fully defined. At this stage, it was normal that there were still many open points, but you had to at least start with a first version. My role now was to continue moderating the meeting. This was more interesting for the IT experts, but from time to time there were questions where the others also took part in the discussion. I found it difficult to maintain my concentration and stay focused. My attention kept jumping to the sore spot on my neck, causing frustration. It became increasingly challenging to articulate and express myself smoothly. The whole meeting became quite dry and bland and we went through field after field in a dull fashion. I would have liked to have livened things up with a joke or two, but I wasn't in the mood for that at the moment. The tension was too high, the pain in my neck too stressful. I was still brand new to the project and this was also an opportunity to showcase my skills to the customer and the project team. Although I was able to score well with my technical skills, my presentation skills were only adequate on this day. I was delighted when the meeting was finally over. I was basically satisfied with the content of the meeting, but I was exhausted.

As it was only afternoon and there was still a mountain of work waiting for us, we drove back to the company's main building. There I sat down in front of my laptop without talking to anyone else. All the project participants were working together in an open-plan office. I had to concentrate hard to block out the other colleagues' conversations and be able to work. In the same way, I had to try to block out the pain in my neck by concentrating. But I only managed this miserably today. I spent the next three hours sitting in front of my laptop, extremely unproductive and tense. The many topics I was supposed to be working on were racing through my head. I couldn't get a clear thought and barely made any progress with my topics.

I also didn't feel like having a coffee and socializing to get to know my new colleagues a little better. I meditated on the toilet for five minutes, but that didn't help much. When I reached my apartment after work, I collapsed on my bed and slept for two hours.

It didn't help, after three weeks I had to abandon the project. With this headache and neck pain, it was impossible for me to survive in this complex situation with new colleagues, new customers and new company processes. I was deeply disappointed in myself. Once again, I had lost my girlfriend and my project due to my constant problem with head and neck pain.

I had serious doubts as to whether I would be able to continue working in my job at all, whether I would be able to afford the loan for the house, whether I would ever find a wife and whether my health would ever improve again.

Worries about the future

I had made an agreement with the couple from whom I had bought the house that they could live in it for another year and a half. In the meantime, they could build their new house and then move straight in.

On October 1, we completed the handover. Everything was in good condition and they kindly gave me some furniture and curtains at a reasonable price. I now went to the house every week to see what was going on. Since I had canceled the project, I had plenty of time.

But every time I reached the house after three quarters of an hour's drive, my mood dampened. The question of what I should do with the house kept popping into my head. I now had a vacant house, a really nice house, a very large and expensive house. But I actually wanted to do something with meditation here. How could that work now that I no longer had a job? I didn't want to move into a huge house at the end of civilization on my own, that much was clear. If I really wanted to hold events here, I would have to convert the attic into a meditation room and rent out the rest of the house at the same time. But how? I didn't have the money for an extension. I didn't even know if I would ever be able to work in my job again and raise enough money to pay off the loan. Taking out another loan in this situation didn't seem like a good idea to me either.

These thoughts and worries choked my throat and kept coming back. My labeling practice suddenly seemed completely ineffective.

I seriously considered whether all this stress with the house was even worth it. Why was I doing this to myself? It was quite a burden. Wouldn't I be better off selling it again and letting go of my dream of being a meditation teacher? Would I feel relieved? But what did I want to do in life instead? Did I still have an alternative plan in my pocket, another good idea?

Was there something else that I wanted in a similar way? Or perhaps it was enough to just continue being an SAP consultant and start a family at some point?

No, that didn't seem to be enough for me, and I couldn't think of anything better. That was the answer that some part of me had ready.

In the end, it was a load off my mind when I found a company that rented the house for its mobile phone technicians as an apartment for fitters. That was a good solution for a start. I could use the rental income to service the loan and had the option of using it myself again in a few years if I wanted to. That gave me some breathing space again.

Back on medication

I had a good family doctor for a while. He was one of the few doctors on my long odyssey who listened attentively and with whom I could talk well. He was able to assess my situation and was also familiar with chronic pain.

To prevent a permanent pain memory from forming again, he prescribed me the painkiller Tramadol, an opioid, in combination with Novalgin painkillers. It was only at this high dosage that I felt any real improvement in the pain. To stabilize me emotionally, he prescribed me the antidepressant Citalopram.

This combination of stronger painkillers showed a real effect on the pain for the first time and reduced the discomfort noticeably. Nevertheless, the pain was still too severe and fluctuated between five and nine on the pain scale, with a maximum of ten. The tablets helped me to stabilize my overall condition somewhat. Attempt number twelve showed some signs of success, but did not bring about a breakthrough.

I hadn't seen a pain specialist since my Kiel days, as fortunately it hadn't been necessary. But now it had escalated again to such an extent that I thought it was worth consulting a proper pain specialist in addition to my GP. I had to try something if meditating was no longer the ultimate measure. It was still essential that I meditated every day, and it often reduced the pain levels significantly. But that simply wasn't enough at the moment.

During pain therapy, I was initially asked to keep a pain diary, which I found helpful. Another MRI scan was ordered with a neurologist to rule out the possibility that I was suffering from a tumor in my head. Of course, I didn't have one.

Then I started neural therapy. Twice a week I was on a drip for an hour and received procaine infusions. Procaine was actually an anesthetic, a local anesthetic. According to the description, it was supposed to influence the stimulus lines of the autonomic nervous system and thus alleviate the pain and reduce the development of inflammation and swelling. The dose of citalopram was also increased slightly. This was trial number 13, which brought a slight improvement.

I also looked for a new orthopaedic surgeon. For the first time, I had the feeling that I had found a good orthopaedic practice. They took an interdisciplinary approach. The doctor was about my age and listened to me attentively when I told him about my long history of neck pain. I had the impression that he was genuinely interested in finding a solution to the problem, not just a standardized treatment, as I had so often experienced. Just the fact that he took my complaints seriously was a great relief.

The doctor examined my mobility, had blood taken and wrote me a referral for an MRI scan. The results were available at my next visit. The MRI scan revealed a small herniated disc between the fifth and sixth cervical vertebrae. The doctor explained to me that it was not always easy to tell where the pain was coming from. There were patients with relatively large herniated discs who had hardly any complaints, and there were patients with small herniated discs who had very severe complaints. Both had to be taken into account in the treatment. He prescribed me physiotherapy with warm mud packs and massages to loosen up the muscles. As my blood values showed a severe vitamin D deficiency, he also prescribed a high dose of this. During physiotherapy, I was first laid on my back for 20 minutes on the warm mud packs and then massaged. The massages were very pleasant and also loosened up my back muscles, but they had no effect on the pain symptoms. The exercises I was shown didn't help either - attempt number 14.

In the meantime, I found out more about spinal injuries. I googled on the internet and attended an information event on surgical options for spinal injuries. Surgery in the neck area in particular was normally only performed in emergencies, for example when symptoms of paralysis occurred. However, so-called PRT injections still represent a promising option, it was said. Under computer tomography, injections with a cortisone-containing anesthetic were injected directly into the vertebrae and intervertebral discs where the problem existed. This was intended to inhibit the inflammation and reduce the pain.

The chances of success were quite high and the risks were manageable. My doctor had already told me about this treatment option in case physiotherapy didn't help, and I started to look into it.

Further treatment search

I was still at a loss and unsure about my new cycle of pain. Maybe this herniated disc in my cervical spine had been the cause of the problem all along? Was this finally the explanation for everything? Maybe they had missed it during the MRI scan when I was 19 years old? Or maybe it had only developed in the last few months?" Anything was possible - and unfortunately also uncertain.

The PRT injections into my cervical spine didn't bring any improvement in my pain and I was disappointed once again, as I had hoped for a lot from it. After all, this was the 15th unsuccessful attempt at treatment.

The next time I visited the orthopaedic practice, they also seemed to be at a loss. This time, a different doctor prescribed a laser measurement of my spine for the purpose of making foot orthoses. The examination was not covered by the health insurance and I paid for it myself. The results showed a slight imbalance between right and left, and I was given insoles of different heights. However, I didn't place much hope in attempt number 16 from the outset.

Over the last few months, I had also been having regular osteopathy treatments. My health insurance company paid a large subsidy on the private prescription and it seemed to help a little, at least in the short term - not entirely in vain attempt number 17.

Parallel to this process, I had received a personal recommendation for a Shiatsu massage master from a friend. Despite my skepticism, I wanted to try it out at least once. He listened carefully to my medical history and took notes.

I then had a shiatsu massage, which was painful. However, I had the impression that such a massage was more effective and loosened hardened muscles. He also showed me various exercises with a tennis ball or a gym noodle. I didn't find the exercises bad and did them regularly at home. I had a total of four or five appointments with the Shiatsu master. But as the treatments were quite expensive at 90 euros per session and there was no improvement, I stopped this therapy attempt number 18.

The same friend, who had also had major problems with head and neck complaints for years, once told me about atlas vertebra treatment. It was usually offered by specially trained osteopaths or chiropractors. As far as I understood it, it was a one-off treatment in which the top cervical vertebra, the atlas vertebra, was brought back into the correct position if it was misaligned. By now I was so weary from the constant, severe pain that I was clutching at straws and wanted to leave no stone unturned. I made an appointment with an osteopath in Hamburg, who I found on the internet and who offered this treatment. After a short medical history interview, he did various mobilization exercises with my cervical spine and neck. He stretched and straightened them and then found my neck to be OK. He couldn't find any misalignment of the atlas vertebrae or any other impairments in terms of mobility. He therefore did not carry out an atlas correction and charged me 100 euros for the one-off treatment. When I woke up the next day, my neck pain had increased many times over. I was sure that this was a result of the treatment. For the next two weeks, I was tormented by this extremely severe pain and was almost driven insane. This was one of the biggest failures and attempt number 19.

The orthopaedist had generally recommended that I continue to strengthen my muscles. So I went swimming once or twice a week and also signed up for Kieser training. Kieser runs fitness studios that specialize in people with physical complaints. At Kieser Training, a training concept was created that took my neck complaints into account. I had regular appointments to train my neck muscles on a computer-controlled machine under the supervision of the staff until they were strong enough for free training. All the exercises on the fitness equipment were tailored to my symptoms and I went twice a week. However, even after months of training, there was no significant improvement that I would have attributed to this - attempt number 20.

Visit to the emergency room

A good friend was doing Reiki and spiritual healing herself. She offered me several intensive sessions with her as she knew that I had been suffering from particularly severe complaints recently. I had already received shorter Reiki treatments from her a few times. It had always helped in the short term and relieved the pain a little. Now, however, I received an intensive treatment and she gave me long Reiki sessions on three consecutive days between Christmas and New Year's Eve. She concentrated particularly on the neck area.

The day after the sessions, the neck pain and headaches had become particularly severe, getting worse and worse and seriously driving me mad. In the end, I was so desperate and complained so much to my parents that they persuaded me to go to the hospital.

They were supposed to check me thoroughly from top to bottom and find out what was wrong with me, at least that was the idea. I didn't have much confidence that this approach was promising. But I had confronted my parents so often with my pain and suffering over the last few months and was so powerless that I gave in to their insistence.

So on the first of January 2017, my mother drove the 100 kilometers to Hamburg, picked me up at home and we registered at the hospital in the emergency room. As it was New Year's Day, there were a lot of injured people and we were told it would take a long time. In the waiting room, I had to get up from my chair every now and then and walk up and down the waiting room because otherwise I couldn't stand the pain. I was on the verge of running amok. Anger and frustration were boiling inside me. I wanted to scream and punch! After three and a half hours of waiting, we were called into a consulting room together. A nurse listened to what I had to say about my complaints and wrote everything down. I asked to be admitted as an inpatient so that I could be checked over. She replied that a doctor would be in shortly and would take care of the treatment.

Again we waited half an hour. When the doctor finally arrived, he told us that he couldn't admit me as an inpatient. As I had already had the severe pain for several months, it was not acute but chronic. For chronic symptoms, I would have to consult my GP and develop a treatment plan with him. He could only give me strong painkillers for acute pain relief.

I was frustrated and resigned, but I had expected something like this. After so many attempts, I had learned not to get my hopes up too high. My mother, however, burst into tears and protested in the strongest possible terms. She vacillated between anger, horror and disbelief that her son, who was almost despairing of his pain, was being denied help. But it didn't help. I was given 800 Ibuprofen and 500 Novalgin.

I took pills home with me, which at least numbed me a

little.

This experience was so upsetting for me that I called in sick during the first week of my new project. Attempt number 21 in the emergency room was a disastrous start to the new year and also to my new, old project.

Luck in misfortune

At least I was lucky enough to be able to work part-time again at my last employer, the industrial and automotive supplier. I coped surprisingly well with the four to five hours a day. I even managed quite a lot in the short time and worked extremely efficiently. I also didn't feel as exhausted after work as I did after an eight-hour day. I still had energy left over for other things. I did a lot of sport and regularly spent time with friends, my niece and my sister.

I was still dependent on strong painkillers, including Tramadol, as lighter painkillers had hardly any effect. But it was good to know that I could still do something and continue to earn money. I even undertook further attempts to get to the bottom of my pain problem medically. My current theory was that there must be a microscopic injury somewhere in the neck area that was constantly irritating the nerve. I paid 600 euros out of my own pocket for an upright MRI scan of the spine. As you were scanned in a standing position, the strain on the spine was different to that in a lying position. It was therefore possible that this scanning method could identify problems that were not visible in the lying position. Minor wear was detected in one of the vertebral joints.

However, it was not very likely that this was causing the pain. Apart from this minor irregularity, this diagnosis did not bring any progress either - attempt number 22.

For almost a year now, I had tried to get the renewed

spiral of pain under control with medical procedures, an extensive sports program and lots of meditation in everyday life. I had spent a lot of time on this, but the result was sobering. I was still in a lot of pain, which severely restricted me in all areas of life.

NO MUD, NO LOTUS - RECOVERY NEEDS PATIENCE

Dhammacari

In March, I went on a 10-day retreat at the Dhammacari Meditation Center near Munich. When I arrived there, I immediately met my good friend Svenja, who wanted to give meditation a try on my recommendation. As the retreats are held in silence, we couldn't talk to each other. Nevertheless, we were happy to meet there and grinned warmly at each other.

Hildegard taught me at this retreat and I was dealing with the usual severe pain, anger and frustration the whole time. I had high hopes for this retreat and expected the pain to finally reduce significantly.

And indeed, after they had accompanied me throughout the retreat, they almost disappeared completely on the last day. However, the joy only lasted a day or two before they returned.

At first I assumed that even a retreat wouldn't be able to help me this time. Now I was really at the end of my tether. What recipe would work now? I had played my last joker.

But then, in the weeks following the retreat, things suddenly got better and better in everyday life. The level of pain slowly but noticeably decreased. After months of being a little heap of misery, my self-confidence slowly grew again and I dared to make plans. I even started dating again and tried Tinder and other dating apps. That had been unthinkable just a few months ago!

New rhythm of life

As the pain level decreased, everything else slowly became easier again. But why was this suddenly the case? It seemed to have something to do with the retreat. Apparently, meditation was still a secret weapon that had pulled me out of the mire again this time. I regained a little more confidence in meditating and in my path, even if the doubt still resonated strongly.

I also had the impression that with the new rhythm of life, working part-time, more free time and lots of time to meditate during the week, I was slowly able to develop more joie de vivre again. This also helped to slowly reduce the pain. I meditated again every day for one to two hours, which was very good for me.

It was a process that lasted for months and more than a year in total until I was back to a low level of pain that I could tolerate without painkillers and that didn't restrict my everyday life too much. Eventually, I felt happier again and regained the self-confidence I had lost.++

Bikram yoga, which I had started a few months ago, also

seemed to help. Once or twice a week, I sweated in temperatures of almost 40 degrees Celsius and practiced the same 26 yoga asanas for 90 minutes. The heat made the muscles and tendons more supple, allowing me to go deeper into the postures.

It was incredibly exhausting and completely drained me. But the next day I felt more energetic and relaxed than usual.

The cause of the evil

Looking back, I kept asking myself how I had ended up in this year-long odyssey. Was it simply a symptom of burnout? Was it all due to a physical injury in the neck region, or a slipped disc, or possibly both?

The thesis that it was a physical cause was supported by the fact that the pain was exacerbated by sleeping. Especially when I wasn't sleeping at home in my waterbed, or when my pillow wasn't the right height for me, the pain was almost unbearable the next day.

The fact that the pain was significantly worse every time the day after strength training, provided I had trained the neck region, also spoke in favor of something physical.

Neck massages also always led to me having severely worsened neck and headaches for several days from the following day.

The fact that the pain almost always worsened when I went through periods of severe stress, such as increased demands at work over a longer period of time, suggested that the cause was psychological.

In the course of my research, I had also delved deeper into all kinds of mental disorders. All in all, my symptoms fitted the description of a so-called somatoform disorder quite well. It causes physical complaints, although often no clear organic cause could be found. Many sufferers were told that they "had nothing". This made them feel misunderstood and they wandered from one doctor to the next. In the long term, this could lead to despair and hopelessness, and often to depression.

Of course, it could also be a combination of physical and psychological factors. Perhaps there really was a physical problem related to the herniated disc that came to light under certain circumstances. If I was reasonably relaxed, perhaps there was enough space in the neck region.

However, if the neck was tense due to psychological factors or the neck region was irritated due to physical activity, there may not have been enough space, leading to friction and irritation of a nerve.

Or was the current pain perhaps simply the harbinger of the next spiritual level, a sign of advancement into deeper spiritual layers and stronger impurities? Meditation can be compared to video games. With each level that you successfully complete, your skills and abilities increase. But your opponents also become stronger and more powerful. I have always found this analogy very fitting. As mindfulness and concentration increase, you can move into deeper levels of the mind and also encounter greater impurities that are challenging even for practiced meditators.

Of all the theories, this one naturally appealed to me the most. However, I rather suspected that in the end - as so often in life - it came down to a conglomeration of many factors.

I knew one thing for sure: I had to take better care of myself in future and stop overextending myself so much. But that was easier said than done.

VIPASSANA MEDITATION HAMBURG - A NEW DEPARTURE

The first introductions

Despite all my doubts in the meantime, meditation had proven to be the best long-term remedy for my pain. Now that I was officially authorized, I therefore decided to give teaching a try. At first, I wanted to wait and see how it would develop and how it would feel.

To do this, I first needed a website. Since I had already designed a website for my friend Michael's meditation center in Portugal, I had some experience with it. So I created a new site with the domain name www.vipassana-hamburg.de. I found a lot of joy in creating something new that had to do with Dhamma. At the same time, I wrote to several yoga studios and asked if they had free studio times when I could use their premises. To my astonishment, several of them got back to me. I finally agreed with Gabi, who ran a studio on the Schanze. She herself taught mother and child classes as well as Kundalini yoga and practiced Vipassana meditation in a different lineage with a teacher from Hamburg.

In April 2017, I started my first classes in her yoga studio. Every Wednesday I gave introductions to Vipassana meditation and then we practiced together. The interest was quite encouraging and every week a few new faces came to the introduction. Even though at first it was rare for anyone to come back or join the meditation regularly, I looked forward to meditating together and sharing with people who had a similar interest.

I enjoyed the introductions and meditating together, and it also gave me new strength. The

Participation in the evenings was based on the Buddhist Dana principle as in Thailand: it was free, but I set up a donation box for those who wanted to support it.

Award in Thailand

In May 2017, I traveled to Chom Thong Monastery again to receive an award. Like many other long-term meditators, I had been nominated for an award as a Buddhist supporter. These awards were given out annually by the Thai District Department of Culture in cooperation with the monasteries, and my teacher Thanat had applied for this for me and around 15 others from our community.

It was a great opportunity to see everyone again. I spent ten days at the monastery with many familiar faces that I had met over the years. This time we didn't meditate in silence, but met for meals together in cafés or went on excursions to Buddhist sites together. It was a great time and I was able to share my first steps in teaching with other junior teachers, which was helpful and exciting.

Encouraged by this journey and a few conversations with other teachers, I now wanted to offer meditation days where people meditated together all day long. I arranged several dates, each on Sundays from 9 am to 5 pm. The interest in the meditation days was also quite high. On my first meditation day, I sat in front of 15 people and gave an introduction to Vipassana meditation based on the four foundations of mindfulness. I explained the theoretical basics, demonstrated mindful bowing and walking meditation and explained what needed to be observed during sitting meditation. New students started with ten minutes of walking meditation and ten minutes of sitting meditation. Then there was a short break, after which the next round followed. We took an hour's lunch break and then continued practicing together all afternoon until 5 pm.

The feedback was largely very positive. It was also nice to see how interested people who had come to the introductory session on Wednesdays a few months ago now signed up for a whole day of meditation. I myself enjoyed this form of teaching. I found it wonderful that after the introduction I was able to spend the whole day practicing with like-minded people. This gave me a relatively large amount of meditation practice in my everyday life and I also had social interaction. At the same time, I found deep meaning in passing on my experiences to others.

My own retreats

As I enjoyed it so much and there was enough interest, I thought about whether I should perhaps organize my own small retreats. As my house, which I now regularly rented out, was empty for a few weeks, I decided to carry out an initial test there.

I asked friends of mine who meditated or were interested in doing so whether they would like to join me on a long weekend for a three-day meditation retreat at my house. In the end, a small but nice group came together. The first participant was Nici, who also offered to do the cooking. I knew her from a small private meditation group where we had met regularly for a few years. The second participant was Aron, my friend of many years. Then Ralle and Jan, my two buddies from Berlin, also took part in the weekend. While Ralle had already visited Thailand and completed a course there, Jan didn't have much meditation experience. It was a very pleasant meditation weekend that everyone enjoyed. I was surprised to discover that it hadn't been as time-consuming and tedious for me as I had feared.

As my house had been rented out again for a longer period in the meantime, I rented a house in Lower Saxony a few weeks later for the first official retreat via airbnb, which offered enough space for 15 people and had a beautiful room with a wooden floor for meditation. The retreat lasted from Friday morning until late Sunday afternoon. Nici again took care of the catering and I myself took care of teaching the twelve participants.

There was a great atmosphere that was both cheerful and relaxed. All the participants were extremely motivated and also helped diligently with the daily household chores. Everything went very smoothly and took very little effort on my part. I enjoyed teaching and seeing the students eagerly practicing in the meditation room. I was amazed at how smoothly it all went.

We then organized two more retreats in the house in Lower Saxony, and each time I didn't feel exhausted after the course, but more alive and full of energy than before. So it all seemed to be good not only for others, but also for myself!

Ceremony in Thailand

I was a little excited because it was a special day for me. I was sitting among about 100 people in the new meditation hall in the international meditation center in the monastery in Chom Thong. Most of them were dressed in white and sat on the floor in a tailor's or heel position. On our left sat about 30 monks, dressed in their orange robes. As every year on the first of October, my teacher Thanat was celebrating his birthday. On this occasion, many long-term meditators, assistants and teachers from all over the world traditionally came to Chom Thong. Many had also arrived earlier, as it was Ajahn Tong's birthday just two weeks earlier. His anniversary was always an occasion for a big celebration with three days of festivities and many thousands of visitors. This time was a good opportunity to catch up with old friends and exchange news - and also to pay tribute to our teacher.

As every year, new meditation teachers in the lineage were also authorized on this occasion and were personally presented with a certificate by the venerable Ajahn Tong in a ceremony. In addition, gold-plated copper Buddhas about one meter high were presented to authorized teachers who opened new Vipassana meditation centers in their respective home countries. A few months earlier, Thanat had asked me if I wanted to expand my teaching activities in the future and open my own center near Hamburg. Although I didn't know exactly what this would ultimately look like, I said yes without hesitation. At the ceremony, I was to receive a Buddha and a sign with the name of the center. There were several large and medium-sized Buddha statues on the altar at the front, as well as some signs that were intended for new centers in Germany, Argentina, Colombia, Mexico and Russia.

Ajahn Tong soon entered the meditation hall and the ceremony could begin. His appearance always ensured that all those present reverently bowed to him three times. Even if you met him on the way, it was Thai custom to put your hands in the prayer position and crouch down so that your head was not higher than the revered abbot. The traditional customs and the display of so much humility, as was customary in Thailand, sometimes seemed a little exaggerated to me. But this could not diminish my own deep reverence for this man.

As in all ceremonies, there were also many Bowing and chanting. First, praises were chanted to the Buddha and then the eight precepts were renewed. On occasions such as this, it was customary for the monks present to be generously provided with monetary donations and other gifts such as new robes. At this very special ceremony, a white cloth ribbon was then also distributed around the room from Ajahn Tong so that the Buddha statues, the monks and those receiving the Buddhas were connected to the ribbon to receive a special blessing.

Finally, I was also called forward, bowed three times to the venerable Ajahn Tong and took the lovingly decorated wooden sign with the golden inscription "Meditation Hamburg Vipassana Center". When he handed it over, he added a golden leaf imprint to the sign. This gave me the official blessing of the lineage for opening a center, so to speak. Afterwards, all the recipients of Buddha's came together at the front, held the white cord and received the chantings specially designed for this purpose.

Afterwards, there was a large food buffet outside the hall. It was nice and warm, the sun was shining and I chatted with friends and acquaintances who had crossed my path here time and again over the past few years. I always enjoyed coming here to the monastery in Chom Thong. It almost felt like a second home. For me, it was a very special day that I will cherish in my memory.

LANDHAUS - WHO DARES, WINS - AND SOMETIMES LOSES

Joy and sorrow

With my new lifestyle and regained self-confidence, I built a meditation and yoga room in the attic of my country house. On the one hand, I wanted to teach Vipassana meditation there myself, and on the other, I wanted to rent the building out as a vacation home to families and groups. The extension involved a large investment, which used up all my savings. I even had to borrow money from my parents. Nevertheless, I thought it was a good idea. This way, I could use my house for occasional weekend courses and at the same time finance it by renting it out.

To finance this project and my living expenses, I looked for a new SAP project in Berlin. I worked full-time again five days a week, two of which were in Berlin. This brought in money to finance the expansion, but it was stressful and demanding.

In fact, after almost two years with a low level of pain and a high quality of life, I suffered another relapse of pain that surprised me in its severity. This time, the trigger was probably the new, stressful project in Berlin and the frequent overnight stays there with my brother on the couch, which my neck didn't like at all. This relapse also meant that I had to abandon the project in Berlin, and again it took months for the pain level to slowly decrease again.

Fortunately, by the time the project was canceled, I had earned enough money to be able to afford the extension and interior design of the house. The meditation and yoga room had become nice and big, so that I could easily accommodate up to 16 people.

The brown floorboard laminate and the large, bright window front with a view of the green back garden and the large, old trees gave the room a beautiful, soft and calm atmosphere. I was pleased with the result.

Now it was time to finish the rest of the house so that I could rent it out as a vacation home to small groups. My bank balance was already in the red and I had to borrow money from my parents again, but they were happy to help me this time too. What great parents I had! They supported me enormously with everything to do with the house and especially with the renovation work. Without their help, I would probably have gone crazy in the pain I was in during the renovation phase.

However, I still had slight doubts about how well the rental would work out. Would anyone really want to go on vacation or spend a weekend in a place with few tourist attractions in the immediate vicinity? I had high hopes for yoga groups who rented the house for small retreats and families with lots of children who wanted to spend a weekend in the countryside.

I spent more or less the whole summer in the house and was constantly busy with some kind of work so that I could get started as quickly as possible. At the end of June 2019, the time had finally come: I was able to welcome the first tenants.

THE FIRST RETREAT IN YOUR OWN HOME - AND HOW IT ALL COMES TOGETHER

The organizer

In the last two weeks before my first retreat in my own home, I was very busy with the preparations. I was in constant contact with my aunt Wiebke to coordinate the meal plan. It was her first time cooking for such a large group and also her first time cooking vegetarian food. I was grateful that she had agreed to take on this part. Otherwise it would have been very difficult with the food. I also had to look through and print out all the teaching materials, answer email inquiries from participants and make a list of everything you need for a retreat like this over several days - from pots and dishes to blankets and meditation cushions.

On August 1, 2019, the time had finally come: I picked up my meditation teacher Thanat and his wife Kathryn from the airport in Hamburg. He would be teaching the retreat, just as he had taught at the retreat with Hildegard where I had met him. It was nice to see my teacher again after a long time. Thanat seemed a little exhausted from the flight from Bulgaria, where the last retreat had taken place. Every year he traveled around the world for three to four months, usually together with his wife, to lead courses and retreats in Europe, Asia and America. This was the first time he had come to the north of Germany. The next day, the first Vipassana retreat in the tradition of Ajahn Tong Sirimangalo began in my house. Every day, my teacher and I sat in the reporting room for five to six hours. The meditators came in one after the other and were given teachings or new tasks, asked questions and were questioned by us about their meditation progress.

I also coordinated everything else that was needed: from toilet paper to missing ingredients for the next lunch. We went shopping and ran errands almost every day. It was quite an extensive program, but I managed it quite well. What was even more amazing was how my teacher managed it all at the age of 77.

Our students practiced diligently and were focused on the task at hand. It was nice to see that the new meditation room was always full and seemed to be really well suited to this function. It also gladdened my heart to see the white-clad meditators sitting in the tall grass in the garden in good weather or walking up and down in walking meditation. For the first time, I really realized that the effort and stress involved in buying the house had been worth it. - If only because it gave me such pleasure to see meditators in my garden and to know that they were on the right path.

Ajahn Tong leaves

On December 12, 2019, I received an email via the newsletter distribution list of the Dhammanikhom Meditation Center that the founder of our lineage, the Most Venerable Ajahn Tong Sirimangalo, had suffered a heart attack and was in intensive care. Coincidentally, my teacher Thanat was also in intensive care due to an ailment of his own. The email asked to practice metta meditation for both of them.

The email made me think. Even though I had never had particularly close contact with Ajahn Tong himself, as the founder of our lineage he was ultimately the reason why I had found my way to meditation. I had great respect for his life's work, and the prospect that his life might be coming to an end caused me to reflect deeply. I thought about how I had come to meditate and how my own teacher had come to meditate. I also realized how much we both benefited from meditation and how Ajahn Tong must have fared in his life. I felt a close bond with my teacher Thanat, so the double message was a bit of a wake-up call.

Two days later, I received another email with the news that the most venerable Ajahn Tong Sirimangalo (Phra Prom Mongkol Vi) had passed away on December 13, 2019 at the age of 96. I had turned 41 on the same day. Fortunately, Thanat's condition had improved again.

I had often seen Ajahn Tong in ceremonies during my stays at the monastery in Chom Thong, but had only exchanged a few words with him over the years. As he didn't speak English, we always communicated through interpreters. Nevertheless, he had a lasting influence on my life, for which I was extremely grateful. The most venerable Ajahn Tong Sirimangalo had ordained at the age of 11. He had spent almost his entire life as a monk and dedicated it to Vipassana meditation.

To honor his life's work, to strengthen the community and also to help him make a gentle and healing transition to a pure state, special chantings were held for 100 days in the Maha Sala, the meditation hall of the main monastery in Chom Thong. Members of the Thai royal family also took part in the ceremonies. Some of the chantings were broadcast via livestream on the monastery's Facebook page. All devotees and practitioners worldwide were invited to attend the daily chantings at the same time, and many meditation centers and groups around the world participated.

I also felt called to respond to this call and organized chanting sessions on several Saturdays. We met in small groups with a few interested practitioners, followed the Facebook broadcast of the chantings from Thailand on the projector and chanted along as best we could. It felt nice to remember our great teacher in this way.

Permanent position

In January 2020, I was offered a permanent position as an SAP in-house consultant with my long-standing client, an industrial and automotive supplier in the Hamburg area. I was very happy about this, as I finally had longer-term planning security.

I felt comfortable in the team and was able to work part-time. This gave me enough time to take care of the rental of the house and the meditation courses alongside my work. This arrangement also gave me the freedom to finish writing this book. These living conditions were an ideal mix for me.

My work was very varied. I sometimes programmed reports and smaller routines myself. But I also provided support, tests and user training, specified new requirements together with the specialist departments and was able to drive innovation. Although I worked part-time, the position gave me enough responsibility and creative freedom. I got on very well with the colleague with whom I worked closely, both in terms of content and personally. Collaboration with colleagues from the specialist departments was also usually uncomplicated and productive. I really enjoyed my job, and as this had not been the case for many years of my professional life, I thought it was a great stroke of luck. After many years of professional odysseys,

I had finally found a good place for me. The house was already very well booked in the first year. It was mostly rented by families or friends with children who could play in the large garden. Sometimes yoga or theater groups also came. I calculated that I would be able to cover the loan in the long term and also make a small profit every year. I was now in a secure financial position. I also had enough time to meditate a lot myself and take care of my meditation courses.

Renewed recovery

More than a year later, I had picked myself up again from the last relapse of pain and recovered quite well. I wasn't completely pain-free, I was still dependent on painkillers, and there were always difficult days when I cursed the world. However, the intensity of the pain was generally at a level that I could cope with, so that I could really enjoy life again. As the pain decreased, the feelings of anger and frustration became less and less frequent.

I continued to meditate a lot in my everyday life, but also pursued my hobbies again and met up with friends regularly. I had also had a partner again for a long time, with whom I was very happy. After many ups and downs, my health, private life and career were looking very positive. My lifestyle finally felt like the stable foundation I had been longing for.

My meditation classes also progressed. In addition to the weekly meditation evenings and monthly meditation days, I now also organized three-day weekend retreats in my home every few months. I also organized a basic course once a year to which I invited guest teachers. Many years after I read the book

"Siddharta", I had realized my wish to teach meditation and had integrated this goal well into my daily life.

But why did I actually want to be a meditation teacher? Why had I continued to pursue this goal, despite all the difficulties and pain that this path had caused me in between? Was it still the curiosity and fascination for the exploration of the mind and the prospect of Buddhist enlightenment as described in the book?

After my snowboarding accident, I had suffered years of physical pain and mental suffering of an intensity that I could not have imagined in the worst hell. The pain tormented me every waking moment, robbing me of positive thoughts, the joy of life and ultimately almost all hope. The worst thing during those years, however, had been the feeling of being at the mercy of others, of having no hope and after all the endless, unsuccessful attempts at therapy, there was no light at the end of the tunnel. I was indescribably grateful that I had escaped this hell again. This experience gave rise to my desire to help other people who might be in a similarly hopeless situation. Vipassana meditation had saved my life. I wanted with all my heart to help other people in the same way - by teaching them to help themselves. That was my motivation; that is my Vipassana.

UNSTABLE CERVICAL SPINE - THE UNEXPLORED DISEASE

The Medical Declaration

In the many years of my illness, I have read a lot: Specialist literature, countless articles, posts on internet forums and books by sufferers. I have visited many different doctors, tried countless different therapies and received many assessments and opinions from different doctors and therapists. After all these years, the information and clues became more and more concentrated, leading me again and again to a specific clinical picture. As very few experts could make such a diagnosis at the time, my self-diagnosis was "unstable cervical spine".

Cervical spine syndrome was only a general description of the complaints in the upper part of the cervical spine. However, it did not allow any conclusions to be drawn about the exact causes of the symptoms. The term unstable cervical spine referred more specifically to the cause of the symptoms.

One of the few, but very good medical textbooks on this topic was the book "Acceleration Injury of the Cervical Spine - Cervical Spine Whiplash" written by Michael Graf, Christian Grill and Hans-Dieter Wedig, published by Steinkopff-Verlag. This comprehensive reference book from 2009 provided an interdisciplinary overview of the state of research in many different studies on the subject of whiplash injuries. In simplified terms, the state of research can be described as follows:

- Diagnosis of chronic whiplash injury with cervical spine instability is hardly possible with current imaging techniques
- Doctors are not trained to recognize the disorder
- Patients often suffer severely from the symptoms, including incapacity to work and subsequent psychological disorders
- Health insurance companies do not recognize

the disorder
- Therapy is only promising to a limited extent; in most cases the symptoms can be alleviated somewhat, but not cured
- Healthcare and legal uncertainty due to lack of recognition of the symptoms

Quote (p.193): *Many whiplash patients have had to give up their social lives, their partnerships and their jobs. Insurance claims are not always at the forefront of their complaints. Often their problems are dismissed as mere allegations or, only slightly better, blamed on the psychological level. It should therefore be the main goal of clinicians and researchers to find ways out of this dilemma.*

Usual things

The causes of an unstable cervical spine could be many and varied. One common cause was whiplash. This happened most frequently in car accidents, but it could also happen in sports accidents or, as in my case, when skiing or snowboarding. The whiplash injury damaged microstructures in the vertebral joints and ligaments that were not visible on normal X-ray, MRI or CT images. These injuries could lead to the cervical spine becoming unstable. This instability could in turn lead to many different complaints. The instability often caused tense, hardened muscles, which then pressed on the nerve pathway to the brain and irritated it. This nerve irritation could cause a whole range of symptoms:

Neck pain and headaches, dizziness, tinnitus, hearing loss,

Gait instability, impaired cognitive performance, word-finding disorders, anxiety and panic disorders.

Quote (p.184): *However, their complaints are not limited to neuropathic pain in the head and neck region; some symptoms originate in the brain. These brain symptoms include dizziness, drowsiness, tinnitus, impaired concentration, attention and memory.*

Apart from dizziness and unsteady gait, I had personally experienced all of these symptoms during the course of my illness.

Other causes could be a genetic predisposition, age-related osteoarthritis or the hereditary disease Ehlers-Danlos syndrome. People affected by Ehlers-Danlos syndrome suffer from weak connective tissue and poor posture in the vertebrae and ligaments. This also led to an unstable cervical spine and could also cause a variety of complaints.

Diagnosis not possible in principle

It was very difficult to diagnose an unstable cervical spine, as in many cases this was not visible at all with today's imaging techniques.

Quote (p.184): *The usual imaging procedures such as computer tomography or magnetic resonance imaging of the brain can only visualize the morphological structures, but not any functional changes in the brain that have triggered the whiplash syndrome.*

To make matters worse, the symptoms were often very complex and overlapped with other diseases. There was little or no research into the symptoms of an unstable cervical spine. A disorder that was

not treated in medical school, was unknown to most doctors and was not recognized by health insurance companies, probably did not exist in our medical system. But that didn't mean that the disease didn't exist and that many people didn't suffer extremely from it.

The symptoms often caused enormous physical and

mental suffering for those affected, combined with a sharp decline in performance. Many became unable to work due to the symptoms and fell into a depressive spiral. In addition, they were not taken seriously by many doctors and did not receive proper treatment for their symptoms. As no physical cause could be found, most doctors quickly suspected a psychological cause, which further unsettled the patients and was of no help.

There was a small community of experts and sufferers who were trying to raise awareness of the disease and call for more research. I also felt that it was very important to research this condition much more intensively, as the people who suffered from it had very severe limitations in their lives and there were not that few people who were involved in a car accident or skiing accident, for example. In the specialist literature, it was assumed that the symptoms remained chronic in around 10 - 20% of whiplash patients.

Therapy also not possible

As if it wasn't bad enough that there was no proper diagnosis, there was also no proper treatment. The studies showed that measures such as physiotherapy or osteopathy often (but not always) provided some relief from chronic symptoms. But this was usually not enough to achieve lasting and fundamental freedom from symptoms.

HAPPY ENDING - MY JOURNEY CONTINUES

Costs and benefits

Now, as a reader, you might naturally ask yourself: was it worth it? All this insane effort for meditating, and then the pain kept coming back and never completely disappeared? There was no redemption, no happy ending, always new setbacks!

The question is justified. I wrote this book over a period of more than ten years. Actually, I had always intended to finish it only when I had completely resolved the pain through meditation. For a while, it looked like it would work. But even after 20 years of intensive meditation, this is still not the case.

The honest answer is that my life used to be so full of difficulties and negative emotions due to the pain and its accompanying symptoms that my own mind felt like a prison. Even today, there are still some pain-related restrictions and occasional lows, but it is now a very worthwhile life for me with many beautiful moments and a healthy level of satisfaction.

If I hadn't discovered Vipassana meditation for myself, I would still be living in pain hell today. I would probably still be suffering from panic attacks and anxiety. And I wouldn't have been able to finish my studies, work as an SAP consultant or have a relationship. I'm pretty sure of that.

Who knows what the future holds. I will probably learn through meditation to recognize the pain and limitations on even deeper levels as part of my life.

On the other hand, I still have the hope that one day I could be completely pain-free. But if not, that will no longer be a drama. Based on my own experience, I am convinced that if you practise Vipassana meditation intensively over several years, you will also notice that negative emotions such as fear, anger and depression tend to become weaker and less frequent and positive feelings such as gratitude, compassion, joy, serenity   and self-confidence increase.

Today I think that it is quite realistic to significantly reduce intense suffering within a few months and years through intensive practice and to noticeably increase joy in life. I think that Vipassana meditation can be an enormous help, especially for conditions such as chronic pain or depression. A complete resolution of such illnesses may require a very long path of practice or may not always be possible. This depends very much on your own karma and also on the type of illness.

Even though I have experienced many frustrations with my medical treatments and meditation has personally helped me more than medication, combining the two has been my model for success in the long term. I would therefore strongly advise not to rely exclusively on meditation or spiritual practices for conditions such as chronic pain and depression, but rather to see them as separate, complementary measures. In any case, you should try to get professional medical and therapeutic help.

Today, after all the back and forth, I feel that I am on exactly the right path for me on the Vipassana path and on my Buddhist path. At the same time, I also continue to use the medical possibilities to improve my health.

Also, if there should be a medical doctor among the readers who is familiar with medical cases like mine and knows about a promising cure I would be pleased to get a tip.

PAIN AS ROCKET FUEL - A VALUABLE HUMAN LIFE

Motivation

You probably know this from your own life: There are the "Towards motivation", and the "away from motivation". In my journey, which you have followed in this book, it was largely a journey with the „away from motivation": away from the pain, away from the anger, away from the frustration, away from the fears, away from the self-doubt. There was probably also a certain "towards" factor, as I had been fascinated by yoga, meditation and Eastern philosophies from an early age. However, the "towards" factor mainly emerged along the way: towards more self-confidence, towards more well-being, towards a more self-determined way of life, towards more compassion and joy.

I would be rather skeptical about the question of whether you can muster the motivation to meditate for two or more hours every day in order to set out on a path towards such an abstract goal as greater well-being, more self-confidence, more compassion. That would be admirable, of course, and there are certainly such cases, but I imagine it would be much more difficult. In a way, it is probably easier with the away-from method if the level of suffering is high enough.

The constant pain, the depressive thoughts, the anxiety and feelings of inferiority, the loneliness and isolation that resulted from my pain and negativity were terrible and almost unbearable. However, the moment I got to know Vipassana meditation and the Dhamma, this pain became my strongest motivation - my rocket fuel!

The pain drove me to persevere to the end of a long, difficult retreat with many strict rules, even though He drove me to meditate extensively every day instead of spending time with friends. He drove me to use my vacation for a retreat instead of going to the beach with friends. He drove me to persevere through difficult projects to save money for another meditation break in Thailand. He drove me to risk buying a house and creating a place for meditation.

On top of that, I didn't have many options when I was in the most severe pain - and I didn't enjoy life much. I didn't have a girlfriend. Not because I didn't want one; I actually longed for a partner. But in my condition, it was simply not possible for me to convince a woman of my worth, let alone maintain a functioning relationship. I still had a relatively large circle of friends for a long time. But with severe pain, the meetings often caused me more frustration than joy.

If you want to dedicate yourself seriously to Vipassana meditation, it takes time. You also have to give up some things in order to make room in your life for regular meditation and retreats. This is easier for someone who already has fewer options and opportunities in life. He or she has to give up less. In terms of Vipassana meditation, a lot of pain (of whatever kind), a lack of options and perspective can even be an advantage and a strong motivation. It supports the person in the practice as soon as positive results appear and the path becomes visible.

In Tibetan Mahayana Buddhism there is the term "Renunciation". Someone who seriously wants to follow the Buddhist path and align their life to it, perhaps as a monk or nun, should first develop renunciation. This is done by practicing renunciation of the negative aspects of the cycle of existence, such as birth, old age, illness, death.

The mind repeatedly becomes aware of not finding and the separation from what is desired in meditation. As a result, the mind turns away from attachment to the comforts of the cycle of existence and eventually longs for liberation from it. Based on my own history, I think someone who has spent a long time in a state of suffering will more easily develop an understanding of it and a motivation for renunciation and liberation.

Even though I could not imagine a life as a monk, this "renunciation spirit" was automatically deeply rooted in me, as I felt the negative aspects of the cycle of existence in every moment of my life for many years. As terrible as this dark phase was for me, I can be grateful to my pain that it led me onto this powerful path and was ultimately the cause of something so positive.

From a Buddhist point of view, a painful life situation can therefore be more beneficial than a pleasant life situation. One is less susceptible to the illusion that the satisfactions of the senses promise lasting happiness. Such a constellation can be an incentive, a motor and a drive to embark on the path of liberation and dhamma and to use one's precious human life in a meaningful way.

FINAL WORD

According to the Buddha's tradition (Palikanon: Majjhima Nikaya 10 - Satipatthana Sutta), there are four benefits of practicing Vipassana meditation:

1. One is mindful while dying and can remember one's positive virtues and meritorious deeds so that the mind is focused on them.
2. After death, one then attains a blissful realm of existence.
3. The seed, the foundation or predisposition to reach the path, the fruit and Nibbana in later lives is laid.
4. Someone who practices vipassana continuously for seven years achieves one of two results. Either he becomes an anagami, a non-returner, the third stage of sainthood. Or he becomes an arahant and attains nibbana in this life with death.

The Buddha also gave five reasons for practicing insight meditation:

1. to purify the mind;
2. to overcome grief and lamentation;
3. to overcome physical and mental pain;
4. to experience the truth of life;
5. to realize Nibbana.

If you have read this book in full, you now know that it might not be enough to take a one-off 15-day meditation course. This of course depends entirely on

your situation. You need to be guided by your own feelings and intuition as to whether this is a viable and right path for you in your situation. You can understand Vipassana meditation more as a long-term liberation path to strengthen positive emotions and reduce negative emotions. I am sure that every hour and every day of meditation brings its own positive results.

There are a few things you should definitely not do as I did. In particular, it is dangerous to conceal medication intake, feelings and conditions from the teacher in a meditation course. The teacher may then not be able to correctly assess your meditation progress and adjust the exercises accordingly.

Through Vipassana meditation and also precisely because of my pain, I have experienced many miracles big and small, experienced a lot of suffering, learned a lot about myself in a number of crises and transformed a lot. I have been able to embark on an exciting journey through life that continues to this day. I can't wait to see where it will take me and what I will experience next.

If you are interested in practicing Vipassana meditation, I recommend taking a meditation course or a retreat. On my website www.vipassana-hamburg.de you will also find links to other centers in the tradition of Ajahn Tong Sirimangalo worldwide. There are currently two other German meditation centers where courses are offered on a permanent basis. You can also meditate at the main monastery in Chom Thong in the Thai province of Chiang Mai.

Basically, you don't have to be a Buddhist to practise Vipassana meditation. It is an exercise that is based on the body and mind and trains the mind. The technique can also be practiced without any religious affiliation and is open to everyone. As it goes back to the Buddha, we teach in his tradition, and there are also certain rituals such as bowing to the Buddha and small ceremonies that are simply part of it.

What I think is extremely important is the metta meditation after the sitting meditation. It has tremendous power to open the heart and you should do it every time after sitting meditation. After a few weeks or months, there should be noticeable changesand improvements if you practice daily.

With this in mind, I would like to conclude this book with a metta meditation.

May I be free from pain and suffering,
May I be happy and content, free from greed, hatred and delusion,
And may I be protected from danger and misfortune.
May I find peace.
May all beings be free from pain and suffering, may all beings be happy and content, free from greed,
Hatred and blindness.
And may all beeings be protected from danger and misfortune.
May all beings find peace.

THANKSGIVING

I hope attentive readers will have read between the lines
how grateful I am to my parents for loving and supporting
me throughout my life.
I hope you will also have sensed how grateful I am,
especially to my teacher Thanat Chindaporn and
I am very grateful to his wife Kathryn that they were able
to teach me the path of Vipassana meditation in a way that
suited me so well, that they always supported me on my
path and constantly encouraged me.
You will also have realized how great my gratitude is to the
most venerable Ajahn Tong
Sirimangalo is that he taught this meditation technique so
impressively and left it as a gift to the world.
I would especially like to thank Hildegard Huber for
bringing Vipassana meditation in our lineage to Germany.
When she started teaching in the 1990s, Vipassana was still
quite unknown in the West and therefore represented
impressive pioneering work.
I would like to sincerely thank all those who also taught and
inspired me as a teacher, all
Phra Ajahn Ofer in front.
I would also like to thank those who have supported me at
courses and retreats in the Hamburg area: Frieda,
Henning, Nicole, and Aron.
I am particularly grateful to my aunt Wiebke supporting
me, together with her late husband Harry
and especially for cooking vegetarian meals for 15 people

for two weeks during my first basic course.
I would also like to thank everyone who accompanied me
part of the way, encouraged me and gave me
support.
I would also like to thank my siblings very much for
their
permanent support, love and care.

People whose Life stories have inspired me:
Buddha, Mahasi Sayadaw, S.N. Goenka, Dalai Lama,
Milarepa, Nanatiloka Bhikkhu, Nelson Mandela, Barack
Obama, Yogananda.